ASTHMA IN CHILDREN

'During the school years
at least 200,000 children will have asthma (in U.K.) and
although the severity of their symptoms will vary,
the quality of control leaves much to be desired.'

Paediatrics in the Seventies.
British Paediatric Association,
1972. Oxford University Press)

Asthma in Children

Natural history, assessment, treatment
and recent advances

EDITED BY

Jan A Kuzemko, MD, FRCP, DCH

Consultant Children's Physician,
Cambridgeshire Area Health Authority (Teaching)
Peterborough, England
Lately, Visiting Professor of Paediatrics,
University of Arkansas, USA

WITH CONTRIBUTIONS FROM

H Amos, MB, PhD

Immunologist, British Industrial Research Association,
Carshalton, Surrey, England

S Bedford, MB, MRCGP

General Practitioner and Research Assistant in Asthma,
Peterborough, England

S R Walker, PhD

Clinical Pharmacologist,
Glaxo Medical Research Laboratory, Middlesex, England

PITMAN MEDICAL

First published 1976
Reprinted 1977

PITMAN MEDICAL PUBLISHING CO LTD
42 Camden Road, Tunbridge Wells,
Kent TN1 2QD

Associated Companies

UNITED KINGDOM
Pitman Publishing Ltd, London
Focal Press Ltd, London

USA
Pitman Publishing Corporation, California
Fearon Publishers Inc, California

AUSTRALIA
Pitman Publishing Pty Ltd, Melbourne

CANADA
Pitman Publishing, Toronto
Copp Clark Publishing, Toronto

EAST AFRICA
Sir Isaac Pitman and Sons Ltd, Nairobi

SOUTH AFRICA
Pitman Publishing Co SA (Pty) Ltd, Johannesburg

NEW ZEALAND
Pitman Publishing NZ Ltd, Wellington

ISBN: 0 272 79400 7

Cat. No. 21 2030 81

Text set in 11/12 pt Photon Imprint,
printed by photolithography, and bound in
Great Britain at The Pitman Press, Bath

Contents

Preface

To be breathless is to be near death. The child with asthma often suffers unnecessarily because this fact is not fully appreciated. He loses countless hours of school work, of play and enjoyment and of sleep—largely because the care of his condition is poor.

Ignorance regarding the natural history of asthma remains deeply ingrained in the minds of many—'he will grow out of it' is an epitaph as common today as it used to be in my student days, and treatment at times assumes an almost patronising attitude. And yet if we are to offer the most effective treatment we must try to understand the causes. Our aim, in this small book is to give an objective outline of asthma in children and point the way towards a more rational and better management the child of today surely deserves.

Each chapter offers a concise account of the relevant aspects of asthma but, inevitably, an occasional overlap occurs. This is intentional.

I would like to thank the many people who have been concerned in bringing this book to fruition. I am especially indebted to Dr P. Ryan, BA, for reading the manuscript through and for helpful suggestions; to Mrs M. Rushford, Librarian, Postgraduate Medical Centre, Peterborough; and Mrs C. Wilson, my secretary. Lastly I thank my long suffering wife for patiently typing the many drafts, and for her forbearance, support and encouragement, without which this book could not have been completed.

I take full responsibility and apologise for any omissions and inadequacies.

Jan A. Kuzemko.

CHAPTER 1

Definition

Jan A. Kuzemko

THE WORD ASTHMA (Greek—breathe hard) has retained its meaning intact through the centuries, although the pathogenesis of the disease remains poorly understood. Thus, in children, asthma must still be defined in clinical and functional terms: '*It is a condition of altered dynamic state of respiratory passages due to the action of diverse stimuli resulting in airways obstruction of varying degree and duration, and reversible partially or completely spontaneously or under treatment.*'

Childhood asthma is a heterogeneous disease. It is familial, meaning that it is inherited by involvement of more than one gene, and environmental factors also play an important role. Indeed, the environmental component is undoubtedly of paramount influence. Many trigger mechanisms provoking episodes of asthma are well understood, but there are others that are not. Despite this, there probably exists a common pathway to explain the clinical features of asthma.

Asthma in children presents in many clinical forms and its degree of severity can be very variable. It may occur in acute attacks, with free intervals lasting from hours to days or even years, or it may occur as a chronic state in which the child has frequent minor and major exacerbations of the disease. Consequently, it may affect lung function to a slight degree or it may develop into a serious handicap resulting in marked disturbance of the life of the child and his family. It is because of its unpredictable course that childhood asthma is poorly understood and difficult to treat, and different views are held regarding its nature and management. Moreover, objective data on asthma in children are scarce and a gread deal of what is available is anecdotal, giving rise to erroneous speculation.

Since much more work has been done on asthma in adults, it is common to find data derived from adults extrapolated to children and a biased interpretation given. It is worth stressing that asthma in children occurs in a pure state and that the degenerative pulmonary diseases of adults are absent; hence, diagnosis and management is of asthma rather than of a symptom complex (chronic bronchitis, emphysema, etc.) often seen in adult practice. Further, the lungs, bronchi and bronchioles actively develop throughout childhood leading to changes in the structure and function.

It follows that a child's lungs must not be regarded as a mirror image of the adult lung. The response to treatment of the asthmatic child is often different from that of an adult and assessment of specific therapy much more accurate. Also, anyone caring for a child must always remember that he deals with a growing patient, as well as the asthma and the patient's family. Hence, not only is a basic objective knowledge of asthma in children essential if the doctor is to do justice to his young patient, but equally important, the interest, enthusiasm and personality of the doctor will have a beneficial effect on both the patient and the family as a whole by encouraging confidence and a better understanding of the disease.

CHAPTER 2

Incidence, Prognosis and Mortality

Jan A. Kuzemko

THE TRUE INCIDENCE of asthma in children remains unknown. Since about half the adult population with asthma and hay fever develop their first symptoms during childhood, study of this subject in children is relevant to its occurrence in adults. In general, up to the age of 15 years, 2 to 3 per cent of boys have asthma and about 1 to 2 per cent of girls. Each year, in England and Wales, well over 8 million children attend school and, with the probable incidence of asthma at this age at about 4 per cent, it can be assumed that 250,000 to 350,000 children will have symptoms of asthma. This assessment does not include pre-school children in whom the incidence of asthma is higher than in the child of 7 to 9 years. Table 2.1 shows the incidence of asthma in children in various areas.

Table 2.1 Incidence of asthma in children in various countries

Authors	Year	Locality	Age (years)	No.	%
Fry[1]	1961	Beckenham, Kent, England	0–10	797	1·5
Graham *et al*[2]	1967	Isle of Wight			2·3
Dawson *et al*[3]		Aberdeen, Scotland	5–16	2,511	4·8
Williams and McNicol[4]	1969	Australia	6–11	30,000	3·7
Morrison-Smith *et al.*[5]	1969–1970	Birmingham, England	5–18	20,958	4·2
Varonier[6]	1970	Switzerland	5–6	4,781	1·69
Rhyne[7]	1971	U.S.A.	Under 10	3,939	6·9
Kuzemko	1974	Peterborough, England	5–11	9,045	4·9

Morrison-Smith[8] studied the incidence of asthma in children at school and showed that in a period of 12 years there was an increase of about 30 per cent. He suggested that environmental factors, especially during the first two years of life, were of great importance in determining the occurrence of atopic disease and hinted that an understanding of these factors at this period of life might lead to a better control of asthma. There are no other studies to support this contention although Fireman[9] in a study of hospital admissions in Pittsburgh, U.S.A. showed that the number of children with asthma admitted to hospital had doubled in recent years and the severity of the disease had increased considerably during the last ten years.

Factors Related to Incidence and Pathogenesis

Family History. Many factors influence the incidence of the disease. A family history of asthma or other manifestations of a hypersensitivity state are often present, varying between 50 and 75 per cent of cases. [12,56,57] The presence of the disease in the mother has much greater significance than disease in the father. Montgomery Smith,[10] in the U.S.A., showed that a child with asthma was twice as likely to have an affected mother than an affected father. This is of interest since more males have asthma than females, and fathers therefore should be affected more than others. Eczema is frequently related, but gastrointestinal allergy and migraine less so. The nature of genetic factors and mode of inheritance is unknown. In a large study of 7,000 twin pairs from Sweden, Edford-Lubs[11] found that allergic diseases had an environmental and a hereditary component and demonstrated that the environmental factor was of much greater importance than had been suggested by any previous study. This was shown by the low concordance rates in the monozygotic twin group (25·3 per cent) and in the dizygotic group (16·1 per cent). The author found that the prevalent rate of allergic disease (asthma, hay fever, or eczema) in the general population was 18 per cent and 40 per cent low penetrance. A distinction between recessive, dominant and multigenic inheritance could not be established. Also, most allergic children were born in families in which neither parent was allergic (67 per cent) or only one parent (30 per cent). The risk of having an affected child from these matings varied from 0·5 to 0·29. In 3 per cent of matings in which both parents were allergic the risk rose to only 0·3.

Allergy. Any material capable of mediating an immunological reaction can initiate a hypersensitivity state. In general, the antigens (allergens) that are of importance in childhood asthma are protein extracts of some form. The common allergens are inhalants, pollens, moulds, bacteria and foods. Atopic eczema occurs at least seven times more commonly in babies fed on whole cow's milk than in breast fed babies. Moreover, Ratner and Silverman[12] reported 59 per cent of children with eczema who subsequently developed asthma and allergic rhinitis. About 5 per cent of children with hay fever will eventually develop asthma. In a seven year follow-up study of 903 college students, Hagy and Settipane[55] found that 6 per cent who developed asthma had previously had allergic rhinitis.

Allergies to food such as cow's milk and egg proteins, related as they are to the respiratory tract, are of importance in the very young child; indeed, cow's milk protein allergy may be the cause of recurrent iron deficiency anaemia, wheezy bronchitis and recurrent otitis media in later childhood.[13]

Sensitivity to house dust is relatively common in children, which is to be expected if it is remembered that house dust contains much organic matter, pollens, dander, moulds and insects, some of which have been fully identified. The house dust mite (*Dermatophagoides pteronyssinus* and *farinae*) is a common sensitiser in children and is associated with humid and damp conditions.[14,39]

Other common allergens are cat, dog and horse dander and, occasionally, aspirin (an idiosyncrasy rather than a hypersensitivity state)[40,42] and antibiotics such as penicillin.

Any child with one form of atopic disease whether it be hay fever, dermatitis, rhinitis or asthma, will often subsequently develop another atopic disorder, e.g. from eczema to asthma. Symptoms in the particular organ can be easily reproduced by very small doses of histamine in the allergic child, but not in normal children.[48] Psychic stimuli can produce similar responses at times. It appears, therefore, that certain children have an inborn predilection to develop atopic diseases, but some as yet unproven environmental factors are also responsible for the acquisition of an atopic state.

Infections. The onset of asthma is often associated with an acute respiratory tract infection. Pearson[15] studied the natural course of asthma in 625 patients. Of these, 393 attributed their first attack to a specific cause. Over 100 stated that it followed an attack of acute bronchitis, 12 after measles, 15 after whooping cough, and 54 after pneumonia or other respiratory infections. The significance of these figures is difficult to interpret because it is possible that such infections only brought out a tendency to develop asthma. A number of authors have tried to demonstrate a relationship between infections and exacerbations of asthma. Viruses such as parainfluenza and respiratory syncytial virus have been reported to cause more exacerbations of asthma than other viruses,[41] and 50 per cent of children eventually developed asthma[16] following an attack of respiratory syncytial virus bronchiolitis.

It is not known whether the allergic child gets more viral infections than the non-allergic. Freeman and Todd[35] showed that wheezing occurred more frequently during respiratory viral illness in the allergic child than in the non-allergic. Berkorvich, Millian and Snyder[17] demonstrated that a third of their children had virus infections at the time of an attack of asthma, while others[36, 38] found concurrent viral infections during exacerbations of asthma, but not all such infections precipitated attacks. Minor and colleagues[37], in a longitudinal study of 16 asthmatic children and their siblings, during a six month period found that children with asthma experienced more viral respiratory infections than their non-asthmatic siblings and when viral infections of an identical nature occurred both in the asthmatic child and his sibling, they took slightly longer to clear up in the asthmatic child. The viruses involved were usually rhinoviruses. Gregg,[18] in a five-year study of respiratory viral infections of children in a London general practice, demonstrated that rhinoviruses were isolated more frequently than any other agent in episodes of asthma in children. He suggested that these viruses were often provocative agents in many children but other host factors were also important. He also found that rhinoviruses and enteroviruses had greater tendency to cause wheezing than other viruses, and that rhinoviruses predominated much more commonly in the child over the age of eight years.

In summary, the relationship of infection to the development of asthma can either be explained as a hypersensitivity reaction to the infecting agent or its products, or alternatively, it is possible that infection is a non-specific precipitating agent of an extrinsic allergic cause of asthma.

Psychosomatic factors. Graham and colleagues[2] found that children with asthma were more often emotionally disturbed and more intelligent than controls, but educational attainments were not greater and the psychiatric disturbance was as common as in any other child with a handicap. Asthma in children is not associated with any specific personality disorder.[19,20] Some attacks of asthma are precipitated by psychological factors[58,60] but it is very rare to find asthma caused exclusively by psychological factors. Mitchell and Dawson[20] in a detailed psychological and psychiatric assessment of 121 asthmatic children found only two with a psychiatric disorder.

There is convincing evidence that although psychosomatic factors can be important in triggering some attacks, there must first exist a somatic substrate for bronchial hyper-reactivity or hyper-irritability before psychosomatic mechanisms can operate.[21,22]

Some children with recurrent severe asthma do appear to have behaviour and emotional disturbances.[63,64] Whether these features are specific for such asthmatic children remains undetermined. Certainly, one cannot identify any definite fault in the mother-child relationship.[65] Mothers of children with asthma do not differ from mothers of children with any other chronic condition.[2] In an Australian investigation,[64] it was suggested that mothers of children with very severe asthma were more anxious and put more restrictions on their children (overprotection) than mothers of a control group. But such findings are surely to be expected from a disease that is life-threatening.

Nevertheless, personal interrelationships within a family setting must have an influence on the course of the child's asthma and there can be little doubt that many attacks are provoked by tensions within the household. In one study,[2] emotional states (fear, excitement, anger) were responsible for about 35 per cent of attacks of asthma. Other factors that can trigger attacks may be associated with laughing, crying, coughing or hyperventilation. The exact way such factors operate in producing bronchospasm remains uncertain.[66]

It is also to be remembered that the majority of published research deals with a very selective group, usually in or attending hospital, i.e. severe asthma, hence any conclusions reached would apply only to such a group and not to the considerably larger proportion of asthmatic children living in a community.

Educational and Social Characteristics. A number of studies have shown that the incidence of asthma in children increases with parental wealth.[2,45] Mitchell and colleagues, on the other hand,[22] found an excess of severe asthma in children of semi- and unskilled manual workers (social classes IV and V) and these children tended to come from large families of four or more children. Pinkerton and Weaver,[52] in an analysis of 206 children with asthma, found sociopathological factors in 44 per cent of those who were resident in special schools but only in 15 per cent admitted to a children's hospital. In two studies,[2,22] the intelligence quotient of asthmatic children was higher than that of the control group. In an Australian study,[63,64] the socioeconomic conditions of the family were found not to be significantly different in children with asthma compared with a control group. However, a study of 1,190 children (6 to 11 years of age) in the United States[59] failed to show any differences between allergic and other children in regard to arithmetic, reading and intelligence tests. The allergic children were less emotionally responsive than the control groups and were found to repress conflict, which produced emotions such as aggression in a significantly higher proportion of cases.

It is possible, yet unproven, that children with asthma are more intelligent than children in the general population, but they do not appear to over-achieve in school work and life careers.

It is common knowledge that children with asthma are good at sedentary occupations such as reading and writing, card playing, jig-saw puzzles, etc. This fact may help to explain to a certain extent the marginally higher intelligence quotients of the asthmatic children observed in some of the studies.

Exercise. Most children with asthma have attacks shortly after physical exertion such as free running[50] or running on a treadmill.[51] Within 3 to 10 minutes of an 8 to 10 minute period of exercise bronchoconstriction occurs, as evidenced by a pulmonary lung function testing, or a frank clinical attack requiring treatment may ensue. The bronchospasm disappears during the next 30 minutes or so. The nature of this bronchoconstriction is uncertain, but it does not appear to be related to mechanical irritation (cold air, dust), hyperventilation, metabolic acidosis or hypocapnia.[43,44] It may, however, be mediated by the involvement of the parasympathetic nervous system.[50,71] Children with eczema alone do not show similar findings.[68]

A very short exercise of one to two minutes duration or early during a more prolonged exercise, the majority of asthmatic and normal children develop bronchodilation,[50,51] which is most likely due to excessive sympathetic activity.[67] There is some evidence that, during exercise, predominantly large bronchi (greater than 2 mm diameter) become obstructed[69,70] but undoubtedly the small airways also become involved during severe exercise and are responsible for the 'air hunger' many children experience.

It has been observed that the majority of children with asthma will develop bronchoconstriction if they exceed a certain threshold of exertion, usually at a heart rate of 150 or so per minute.[51,72]

The exercise test forms the basis of the Bronchial Lability Index for assessing asthma, as devised by R. S. Jones,[23] and is discussed further on pages 33 to 35.

Pollution and Climate. It is not clear whether pollution and the mobility of the population because of exposure to different climatic conditions have any role to play in the development of asthma. Ribon and colleagues,[24] in a statistical analysis of asthma in children and its occurrence in relation to weather and air pollution, showed an increase in the percentage of visits and admissions of children to hospital and clinics during the autumn months. In Queensland, Australia, it was shown that not only in autumn was there a rise of admissions but also in the spring. The nature of the factors concerned was undetermined.[61] No significant relationship was found in the daily air pollution averages but there was a tendency for change in temperature to be related to changes in the number of asthma consultations. Smoke and wind direction may act as non-specific irritating factors in provoking attacks.[54] Breathing cold air alone may induce bronchospasm, possibly through the efferent cholinergic pathways in the upper airways.[62] A study of the effects of humidity in 18 children in an air-conditioned chamber failed to show any definite exacerbations.[73] A six-month study of 105 children with asthma living in the South of France demonstrated that extremes of environmental temperatures had bronchoconstrictive effects on the airways.[74] It would seem, therefore, that environmental factors may be important in exacerbation of asthma and very likely these factors operate together rather than alone.

Table 2.2 Mortality from asthma

Authors	Year	No.	Follow up (years)	Death rate %
Rackemann & Edwards[25]	1952	688	20	1
Barr and Logan[26]	1964	324	22	1
Buffum & Settipane[27]	1966	136	20	2·5
Leveque & colleagues[28]	1969	94	5	4
Viallatte & Paupe[29]	1971	231	5–14	0·45

Mortality. The mortality rate varies between 1 and 4 per cent, which is shown in Table 2.2. The number of deaths in England and Wales from asthma per 100,000 children aged 5 to 14 is between 25 and 35 each year, excluding the years 1963–1966 when the annual number of deaths attributed to asthma increased.[75] Several reasons for this change in mortality have been discussed extensively by Speizer, Doll, Heaf, Strang, and others.[30,46,47] Since 1967, the death rate from asthma in Britain has declined to the pre-1960 years.[75]

Prognosis. The knowledge of factors affecting prognosis remains incomplete. A review of the literature shows that two factors have been thought to be of prognostic significance, namely the age of onset and the relationship to allergy. It has been found that the majority of children develop asthma during the first two years of life and their prognosis is much worse than those children who develop asthma later in childhood.[3,49] The presence of atopic disease such as eczema or hay fever signifies a poorer outlook.[34] Also, the more severe the symptoms in early childhood the more likely it is that asthma will continue into adulthood.

Table 2.3 Prognosis of childhood asthma

Authors	Year	Place	No.	Symptom (free)	Asthma % Improved	Asthma % Unchanged
Rackemann & Edwards[25]	1952	Massachusetts	499	31	56	13
Ryssing & Fleusborg[31]	1963	Copenhagen	442	37	9	54
Aas[32]	1963	Oslo	174	44	17	39
Kraepelien[33]	1963	Stockholm	528	29	65	6
Leveque & colleagues[28]	1969	Paris	94	31	43	22
Viallatte & Paupe[29]	1971	Paris	221	57	33	10
Barr & Logan[26]	1964		336	52	No details	

Table 2.3 shows the long-term prospects for the asthmatic child. On average, observations have been made between 5 to 20 years. Engstrom, Kraepelien and Noren[33,53] found that in a group of 528 asthmatic children the long-term outlook was less favourable than was generally claimed. Over a 13-year period of observations, 29 per cent of the individuals were symptom free, 70 per cent still had asthma but were considerably improved, 4·9 per cent remained unchanged, 1·1 per cent deteriorated, and 0·4 per cent died.

There is some evidence that in the child with predominantly allergic asthma, early hyposensitisation may lead to better prognosis.[34,29] However, there are few other data to support or disprove this contention. One can only speculate that with the discovery of sodium cromoglycate and steroid aerosols, the outlook for the asthmatic child who is adequately assessed and treated will be very much brighter than was the outlook for his predecessors.

References

1. Fry, J. (1961) *The Catarrhal Child.* Oxford: Butterworths.
2. Graham, P. J., Rutter, M. L., Yule, W. and Pless, I. B. (1967) Childhood asthma; a psychosomatic disorder? Some epidemiological considerations. *British Journal of Preventure and Social Medicine*, **21,** 78.
3. Dawson, B., Horobin, G., Illsley, R., Mitchel, R. (1969) A survey of childhood asthma in Aberdeen. *Lancet*, **1,** 827.
4. Williams, H. and McNicol, K. N. (1969) Prevalence, natural history and relationship of wheezy bronchitis and asthma in children. An epidemiological study. *British Medical Journal*, **2,** 321.
5. Morrison-Smith, J., Harding, L. K. and Cumming, G. (1971) The changing prevalence of asthma in school children. *Clinical Allergy*, **1,** 57.
6. Varonier, H. S. (1970) Prevalence of allergy among children and adolescents in Geneva, Switzerland. *Respration*, **27,** 115.
7. Rhyne, M. B. (1974) Incidence of atopic disease. *Medical Clinics* of N. America, 58, 1, p.5.
8. Morrison-Smith, J. (1974) Studies of the prevalence of asthma in childhood. Abstract, 9th European Congress of Allergology and Clinical Immunology, London.
9. Fireman, P. (1971) A review of asthma admissions and deaths at the Children's Hospital of Pittsburgh from 1935 to 1968. *Journal of Allergy*, **46,** 257.
10. Montgomery Smith, J. (1974) Incidence of atopic disease. Medical Clinics of N. America, 58, 1, p. 10.
11. Edford-Lubs, M. L. (1971) Allergy in 7,000 twin pairs. *Acta Allergologica*, **26,** 249.
12. Ratner, B and Silverman, D. A. (1953) Critical analysis of the hereditary concept of allergy. *Journal of Allergy*, **24,** 371.
13. Gerrard, J. W. (1966) Familial recurrent rhinorrhea and bronchitis due to cow's milk. *Journal of the American Medical Association*, **198,** 605.
14. Spieksma, F. (1970) Biological aspects of the house dust mite (*Dermatophagoides pteronyssinus*) in relation to house dust atrophy. *Clinical Experimental Immunology*, **6,** 61.
15. Pearson, R. S. B. (1958) Natural history of asthma. *Acta Allergologica*, **12,** 277.
16. Zweiman, B., Schoenwelter, W. F., and Hildreth, E. A. (1966) The relationship between bronchiolitis and allergic asthma. A prospective study with allergy evaluation. *Journal of Allergy*, **37,** 48.

17. Berkovich, S., Millian, S. J. and Snyder, R. D., (1970). The association of viral and mycoplasma infections with recurrence of wheezing in the asthmatic child. *Annals of Allergy*, **28,** 43.
18. Gregg, I., Horn, M. and Yelland, S. (1974) The role of viral infection in asthma and bronchitis. Abstract, 9th European Congress of Allergology and Clinical Immunology, London.
19. Leigh, D. and Marley, E. (1967) *Bronchial Asthma: a Genetic Population and Psychiatric Study.* Oxford: Pergamon Press.
20. Mitchell, R.G. and Dawson, B. (1973) Educational and social characteristics in children with asthma. *Archives of Disease in Childhood*, **48,** 467.
21. Feingold, B. F., Singer, M. T., Freeman, E. H. and Deskins, A. (1966) Psychological variables in allergic disease: a critical appraisal of methodology. *Journal of Allergy*, **38,** 143.
22. Freeman, E. H., Feingold, B. F., Schlesinger, K. and Gorman, F. J., (1964) Psychological variables in allergic disorders: a review. *Psychosomatic Medicine*, **26,** 543.
23. Jones, R. S. (1966) Assessment of respiratory function in the asthmatic child. *British Medical Journal*, **2,** 972.
24. Ribon, A., Glasser, M. and Subhivorseth, N. (1972) Bronchial asthma in children and its occurrence in relation to weather and air pollution. *Annals of Allergy*, **2,** 276.
25. Rackemann, F. H. and Edwards, M. C. (1952) Asthma in childhood. Follow up study of 688 patients after intervals of 20 years. *New England Journal of Medicine*, **246,** 815 and 858.
26. Barr, L. W. and Logan, G. B., (1964) Prognosis of children having asthma. *Pediatrics*, **34,** 856.
27. Buffum, W. P. and Settipane, G. A. (1966) Prognosis of asthma in childhood. *American Journal of Diseases of Childhood*, **112,** 214.
28. Leveque, B., Jean, R., Benoit, M. R., Cloup, I., Mischler, J. and Marie, J. (1969) Evolution, pronostic eloigne et retenissement social de la maladie asthmatique de l'enfant. *Annales de Pediatire*, **45,** 1459.
29. Villatte, J. and Paupe, J. (1971) Course and prognosis of asthma in children. Abstracts, 8th European Congress of Allergology and Clinical Immunology, Paris.
30. Speizer, F. E., Doll, R., Heaf, P., and Strang, L. B. (1968) Investigation into the use of drugs preceding death form asthma. *British Medical Journal*, **1,** 339.
31. Ryssing, E. and Fleusborg, E. W. (1963) Prognosis after puberty for 442 asthmatic children examined and treated on specific allergologic principles. *Acta Paediatrica* (Uppsala), **52,** 97, 100.
32. Aas, K. (1963) Prognosis for allergic children. *Acta Paediatrica Scandinavica, Supplement* 140, **87,** 81.
33. Kraepelien S. (1964) Prognosis of asthma in childhood with special reference to pulmonary function and the value of specific hyposensitisation. *Acta Paediatica Scandinavica Supplement*, 140, **87.**
34. Johnstone, D. E. and Dutton, A. (1968) Value of hyposensitisation for asthma in children—a 14 year study. *Pediatrics*, **42,** 793.
35. Freeman, G. L. and Todd, R. H. (1962) The role of allergy in viral respiratory tract infections. *American Journal of Diseases of Childhood*, **104,** 330.
36. Minor, T. E., Dick, E. C. and Demeo, A. N. (1974) Viruses as precipitants of asthmatic attacks in children. *Journal of the American Medical Association*, **227**, 292.
37. Minor, T. E., Baker, J. W., Dick, E. C., Demeo, A. N., Oulette, J. J., Cohen, M. and Reed, C. E. (1974) Greater frequency of viral respiratory infections in asthmatic children as compared with their non-asthmatic siblings. *Pediatrics*, **4,** 472.
38. Eisen, A. H. (1969) The role of infection in allergic disease. Pediatric Clinics of North America, **16,** 67.
39. Maunsell, K., Wraith, D. G. and Cunnington, A. M. (1968) Mites and house dust allergy in bronchial asthma. *Lancet*, **1,** 1267.

40. Yunginger, J. W. O'Connell, E. J. and Logan, G. B. (1973) Aspirin induced asthma in children. *Journal of Pediatrics*, **82,** 218.
41. McIntosh, K., Ellis, F. E., Hoffman, S. L., Tillinghast, L. G., Eller, J. J. and Fulginiti, V. A. (1973). Association of viral and bacterial respiratory infections with exacerbations of wheezing in young asthmatic children. *Journal of Pediatrics*, **82,** 578
42. Falliers, C. J. (1972) Late-onset asthma linked to aspirin sensitivity. *Journal of the American Medical Association*, **221,** 244.
43. Cohen, A. A. and Hale, F. C. (1965) Comparative effects of isoproterenol aerosols on airway resistance in obstructive pulmonary diseases. *American Journal of Medical Science*, **249,** 309.
44. Vasallo, C. L., Gee, J. B. L., and Domm, B. M. (1972) Exercise-induced asthma: observations regarding hypocapnia and acidosis. *American Review of Respiratory Diseases*, **105,** 42.
45. Freeman, G. L. and Johnson, S. (1964) Allergic diseases in adolescents. *American Journal of Diseases of Childhood*, **107,** 549.
46. Gandevia B. (1967) Pressurized aerosols in asthma. *British Medical Journal*, **2,** 441.
47. Richards, W. and Patrick, J. R. (1965) Death from asthma in children. *American Journal of Diseases of Childhood*, **110,** 4.
48. Szentivanyi, A. and Fishel, C. W. (1966) The chemical mediators of the allergic response to the reactivity of their target cells. In *Pathogenese und Therapie Allergischer Reactionen* (Ed. G. Filipp) Stuttgard, Germany: Grundlegenforschung und Klinik Verlag.
49. Williams, H. and McNicol, K. N. (1969) Prevalence, natural history and relationship between bronchitis and asthma in children. Epidemiological study. *British Medical Journal*, **4,** 321.
50. Jones, R. S., Buston, M. H. and Wharton, M. J., (1962) The effect of exercise on ventilatory function in the child with asthma. *British Journal of Diseases of the Chest*, **56,** 78.
51. Silverman, M. and Anderson, S. D. (1972) Standardization of exercise tests in asthmatic children. *Archives of Disease in Childhood*, **47,** 882.
52. Pinkerton, P. and Weaver, C. (1970) Childhood Asthma. In *Modern Trends in Psychosomatic Medicine*, 2 (Ed. O. W. Hill). London: Butterworths, p. 95.
53. Kraepelien, S. (1950) The frequency of bronchial asthma in Swedish school children. *Acta Paediatrica (Uppsala)*, **43,** Suppl. 100, p. 149.
54. Spotnitz, M. (1965) Significance of Yokohama asthma. *American Review of Recipratory Diseases*, **92,** 371.
55. Hagy, H. W. and Settipane, G. A. (1975) Risks of developing asthma and allergic rhinitis: A 7 year follow-up study of 903 college students. *Journal of Allergy and Clinical Immunology*, **55,** 2, 124.
56. Van Arsdel, P. P. and Motulski, A. G. (1959). Frequency and hereditability of asthma and allergic rhinitis in college students. *Acta genetica et statistica medica (Basel)*, **9,** 101.
57. Cohen, C. (1974) Genetic aspects of allergy. *Medical Clinics of N. America*, 58, 25.
58. Graham, P. and Rutter, M. (1970) *Education, Health and Behaviour*. (Ed. M. Rutter, J. Tizard and K. Whitmore.) London: Longman, p. 309–27.
59. Rawls, D. J., Rawls, J. R. and Wade Harrison, C. (1971) An investigation of six to eleven year old children with allergic disorders. *Journal of Consulting and Clinical Psychology*, **36,** 2, 260.
60. McLean, J. A. and Ching, A. Y. T. (1973) Follow-up study of relationships between family situations and bronchial asthma in children. *Journal of the American Academy of Child Psychology*, **12,** 142.
61. Derrick, E. H. and Szymanski, S. (1967) The relation of the seasonal variation of asthma to weather; an Australian-wide survey. *Australian Paediatric Journal*, **3,** 82.
62. Simonsson, B. G., Jacobs, F. M. and Nadel, J. H. (1967) Role of autonomic nervous system and the cough reflex in the increased responsiveness of airways in patients with

obstructive airway disease. *Journal of Clinical Investigation*, **46,** 1812.
63. McNicol, K. N. and Williams, H. E. (1973) Spectrum of asthma in children I. Clinical and physiological components. *British Medical Journal*, **4,** 7.
64. McNicol, K. N., Williams, H. E., Allen, J. and McAndrew, I. (1973) Spectrum of asthma in children, III. Psychological and social components. *British Medical Journal*, **4,** 16.
65. Miklich, D. R., Rewey, H. H. Weiss, J. H. and Kolton, S. (1973) A preliminary investigation of psychophysiological responses to stress among different sub-groups of asthmatic children. *Journal of Psychosomatic Research*, **17,** 1.
66. Khan, A. V. (1973) Psychosomatic aspects of asthma. *Psychosomatics*, **14,** 195.
67. Griffiths, J., Leung, F. Y., Grzybowski, S. and Chan-Yeung, M. M. W. (1972) Sequential estimation of plasma catecholamines in exercise-induced asthma. *Chest*, **62,** 527.
68. König, P and Godfrey, S. (1973) Prevalence of exercise-induced bronchial lability in families of children with asthma. *Archives of Diseases of Childhood*, **48,** 513.
69. Cropp, G. J. A. (1975) Relative sensitivity of different pulmonary function tests in the evaluation of exercise induced asthma. *Pediatrics* (Suppl.), **56,** 860.
70. Mildon, A., Leroux, M., Hutcheon, M and Zamel, N. The site of airways obstruction in exercise-induced asthma. *American Review of Respiratory Diseases*, **110,** 409.
71. Simonsson, B. G., Skoogh, B. E. and Ekstrom-Jodel, B. (1972) Exercise-induced airways constriction. *Thoras*, **27,** 169.
72. Katz, R. M., Whipp, B. J., Heimlich, E. M. and Wassermann, K. (1971) Exercise-induced bronchospasm, ventilation and blood gases in asthmatic children. *Journal of Allergy*, **47,** 148.
73. Fontana, V., Holt, L. E. and Mainland, D. (1966) Effectiveness of hyposensitization therapy in ragweed hay fever in children. *Journal of the American Medical Association*, **195,** 985.
74. Charpin, J., Boutin, C., Arnaud, A., Delgove, P. and Orehek J. (1975) Environment and Respiratory Allergic Diseases. *Allergy 1974* Proceedings of 9th European Congress of Allergology and Clinical Immunology (Ed. M. A. Ganderton and A. W. Frankland) London: Pitman Medical.
75. Standing Medical Advisory Committee for the Central Health Services Council. (1973) *Deaths from Asthma*. Dept. of Health and Social Security. London: H.M.S.O.

CHAPTER 3

Physiology and Pathology of the Lung

Jan A. Kuzemko

THE BASIC FUNCTION of the lungs is to exchange gases between the blood in the lung capillaries and the air in the alveoli, providing oxygen for the energy of vital functions, and removing excess carbon dioxide. The degree of gaseous exchange in any child varies according to his age. Disturbances in gas exchange may lead to ineffective oxygenation of various tissues and organs, and retention of carbon dioxide with resultant respiratory and subsequently metabolic, acidosis. The exchange of gases occurs across a delicate membrane separating the air in the periperal lung units from the capillary blood bed. The exchange depends on normal transport of air in both directions in the respiratory passages and of normal active transport across the membrane.

Air that is inhaled through the trachea is distributed into the left and right bronchi. The left and right main bronchi sub-divide into smaller bronchi serving different lobes and segments of the lung (0·5 cm diameter or so). These subsequently divide into yet smaller bronchi and bronchioles. The bronchioles have a diameter of approximately 0·5 mm. Each divides into two respiratory bronchioles of about 0·25 mm diameter, which subdivide into alveolar ducts of 0·2 mm diameter. The number of alveoli in a normal lung is approximately 300,000 with an estimated total surface area of 80 m^2.

The respiratory tract is lined with an epithelium, the basement membrane of which rests on a network of reticular and collagenous elastic fibres and a layer of smooth muscle forming the lamina propria. The lamina propria contains capillaries, lymphatics and nerves. Large numbers of lymphocytes and associated immunoglobulins are present, which represent important sources of local antigen-antibody reactions.[1] The bronchial wall contains an abundant number of mast cells. Salvato[11] showed that lung biopsies taken from patients during an attack of asthma, contained a diminished number of intact mast cells in the bronchioles and numerous cells that were disrupted and degranulated. In addition, granules were found in the surrounding tissues. These granules contain pharmacologically active substances such as histamine and heparin. The lungs are richer in histamine than any other human organ.[2] The other known mediator is the slow reacting substance of anaphylaxis (SRS–A). Its source is unknown but it is probably associated with mast cell degranulation. The nature of other mediators, e.g. prostaglandins, awaits further investigation but may be important.[25,26] Histamine and SRS–A induce contraction of the smooth muscle, hence once released into airways they can cause bronchospasm. Since they are both irritant mediators, inflammatory changes commonly result (oedema, hypersecretion of mucus) and lead to obstruction of the air flow.

The mucosal lining of the air passages contains ciliated epithelium as far down as the peripheral bronchioles. The cilia are covered by mucus and beat towards the external orifice, thus removing any secretions or foreign material. The mucus flow rate is 10 to 15 mm a minute in the subglottic space.[3] There is evidence that the mucus is both bactericidal and virucidal. The mechanism controlling the ciliary activity is unknown but it appears to be under nervous control. Acetycholine is present in nerve and mucosal tissues and may be responsible for some of the ciliary action. It is probable that serotonin also plays a part.[3,4]

Bronchial secretions are produced by goblet cells sited in the surface epithelium and by the serous and mucus glands deep in the bronchial wall. The goblet cells secrete a watery material whereas the serous and mucus glands produce a tenacious substance. The goblet cells are stimulated by direct action and are not under the control of the autonomic nervous system with the cholinergic system stimulating increased glandular secretion. Excessive secretions can also be evoked by histamine and bradykinin. Bronchial glands produce secretions such as mucopolysaccharides, glycoproteins, etc., but the relationship between these is not yet clear.[5]

Smooth muscle is found throughout the entire length of the air passages and even in the walls of the peripheral alveolar ducts. In the large bronchi it is situated posteriorly between the rings of cartilage. In the small bronchi and bronchioles it is arranged in a spiral pattern and is increased in density compared with the size of the lumen. Smooth muscle cells are situated in direct contact with nerve endings of the sympathetic and parasympathetic nervous systems. Parasympathetic nerve stimulation results in bronchoconstriction and sympathetic in bronchodilatation.

The normal flow of air and normal tone depend on the existence of a balanced interaction of the two components of the autonomic nervous system, and tissue receptors acting on them. The stimuli are transmitted by various chemical mediators acting on the receptors which are sensitive to them, such as the alpha and beta receptors.

Szentivanyi[15] proposed that an individual with bronchial asthma behaves as if his beta-adrenoreceptors were partly blocked, i.e. he has impared adenyl cyclase response to catecholamines. The theory has been supported by some recent scientific observations: for instance, Lichtenstein and Gillespie[16] studying leucocytes, have shown that drugs that increase intracellular cyclic AMP concentration, e.g. theophylline, inhibit histamine release which, once released, prevents its own further formation; and Parker and colleagues[17,18] studying lymphocytes and leucocytes, showed that such cells in asthmatic patients had significantly lower levels of cyclic AMP than did controls, that the levels were lowest during exacerbations of asthma, and that the cells responded normally to prostaglandin E_1 which activates adenyl cyclase by a mechanism not involving beta-adrenoreceptors.

In non-asthmatic subjects, blockade of beta-receptors does not cause bronchial constriction.[23] In asthmatic individuals, however, beta-blockade results in bronchoconstriction.[24] It is suggestive thus that the asthmatic person has increased beta-adrenergic activity which allows unopposed the effects of any constrictor stimuli on the smooth muscle (Table 3.1).

Table 3.1 Smooth muscle tonicity

Dilator Stimuli	*Constrictor Stimuli*
Prostaglandin E	Histamine
Beta-adrenergic	SRS–A
	Bradykinin
	Prostaglandin $F_{2\alpha}$
	Parasympathetic
	α adrenergic

Parasympathetic nerves act through acetycholine, and the sympathetic nerve stimuli are mediated by catecholamines. There also exist short circuit reflex pathways that may cause bronchoconstriction when irritating substances such as gases or cold air are inhaled. There is also evidence that there are receptors in the nose and nasopharynx that may cause a bronchoconstriction reflex.[6] In addition, bronchi may become constricted following hypoxia or hypercapnia.

The patency of the alveoli depends on a surfactant which lines them and this consists of lipoproteins that are rich in lecithin. Thus, any factor interfering with sufactant production may result in instability of the pulmonary structure leading to aveolar collapse.

Sites of airway obstruction. In children with severe asthma, airway resistance is increased and the maximum expiratory flow is decreased. This implies that both large and small airways are narrowed. Constriction of smaller airways is probably more common in children although the site of the airway obstruction may be variable, depending on the aetiology of a particular attack.[9,19,20] These observations suggest that smooth muscle response to noxious stimuli can vary in different parts of the airway. Thus, in a child with severe asthma any test measuring expiratory flow would be markedly reduced. Following therapy, changes may revert completely to normal, although abnormalities may often be shown when sensitive tests such as closing volume or frequency dependence of compliance,[21,22] are used.

Inspired air can be distributed in an uneven way in asthma, even in the patient with mild disease, and can result in poor ventilation—perfusion of the inspired gas in some areas of the lungs. If large areas become affected arterial hypoxaemia will occur. For the same reason, inhaled bronchodilator agents may reach only well-ventilated zones, providing only a marginal increase in ventilation that is of little therapeutic value. The arterial PCO_2 in children during an attack of asthma is usually normal or decreased because of hyperventilation. Hence, an increased arterial PCO_2 indicates imminent ventilatory failure, and a need for urgent intensive treatment.

Asthma, therefore, is not only associated with bronchospasm, but also with an increase in the amount of gas retained in the lungs. This can easily be confirmed by measuring the expiratory volume in the first second (reduced), residual volume (increased) and the vital capacity (reduced). Such findings indicate that the small airways between the bronchi and the alveoli must be extremely narrowed or completely blocked before expiration begins.

During an attack of asthma airway closure occurs at a high lung volume. In addition to bronchoconstriction, intraluminal factors such as mucus and oedema, also operate, leading to complete obstruction of the small airways. The mucus membrane plays a part in such obstruction as it is thrown into folds projecting into the lumen.[10]

The child, therefore, breathing at high lung volume has to work very hard to inspire because his respiratory muscles are at some mechanical disadvantage. In fact, he finds it more difficult to inspire than to expire. As the severity of asthma increases, the child's cardiac output and oxygen consumption rise and, due to the negative pressure within the chest, there is an increase of the transluminal pressure on the left atrium and the pulmonary circulation. Such a course of events, at a time when the gas exchange and the cardiac output are already seriously compromised, results in a fall of the minute ventilation and leads to distressed breathing.

Pathology. Some of the above observations can be confirmed at post mortem in children who have died during an acute attack of asthma. The lungs are distended and small bronchi up to 1 mm in diameter are usually obstructed with thick plugs of mucus.[12] Microscopy of the wall shows an increase in the number of goblet cells and mucus glands and some shedding of the superficial epithelium. The basement membrane is thick, and large numbers of eosinophils and lymphocytes are present in the mucus and in the wall of the bronchus. The very small bronchi often show squamous metaplasia as well as thickening of the basement membrane. The bronchial muscle is hypertrophied and areas of infection either in the alveoli or in the tissues may be present.[7,8] Bronchial biopsy of the asthmatic lung usually shows subepithelial infiltrations with eosinophils, a feature that distinguishes asthma from chronic bronchitis.[11,13,14]

Suggestions for further reading

Bouhuys, A. (1974) *Breathing, Physiology, Environment and Lung Disease.* New York: Grure and Stratton.

Liebow, A. and Smith, D. E. (Ed.) (1968) *The Lung*. Baltimore: Williams and Williams.

Scarpelli, E. M., Auld, P. A. M. and Goldman, H. A. (Ed.) (1973) *Pediatric Pulmonary Physiology and Disease*. Philadelphia: Lea and Febiger.

References

1. McCarter, J. H. and Vazgnez, J. J. (1966) The bronchial basement membrane in asthma. *Archives of Pathology (Chicago)*, **82,** 328.
2. Stone, J. L., Merrill, J. M. and Meneely, G. R. (1955) Distribution of histamine in human tissues. *Federation Proceedings*, 14, 147.
3. Van, AsA. and Webster, I. (1972) The organisation of ciliary activity and mucus transport in pulmonary airways. *South African Medicine*, **46,** 347.
4. Burn, J. H. (1958) The antihistaminic compounds. *British Medical Journal*, **2,** 845.
5. Reid, L. (1968) Bronchial mucus production in health and disease. In *The Lung* (Ed. Liebow A. and Smith D. E.) Baltimore: Williams and Williams.
6. Kaufman, J. and Wright, G. W. (1969) The effect of nasal and nasopharyngeal irritation on airway resistance in man. *American Review of Respiratory Disease*, **100,** 626.
7. Dunnill, M.S. (1960) The anthology of asthma with special reference to changes in the bronchial mucosa. *Journal of Clinical Pathology*, **13,** 27.
8. Dunnill, M. S., Masserella, G. R. and Anderson, J. A. (1969) A comparison of the quantative anatomy of the bronchi in normal subjects, in status asthmaticus, in chronic bronchitis and in emphysema. *Thoras*, **24,** 176.
9. Messer, J. W., Peters, G. A. and Bennett, W. A. (1960) Causes of death and pathological findings in 304 cases of bronchial asthma. *Diseases of the Chest*, **38,** 616.
10. Horsfield, K. (1974) The relation between structure and function in the airways of the lung. *British Journal of Diseases of the Chest*, **68,** 145.
11. Salvato, G. (1961) Mast cells in bronchial connective tissue in man. *International Archives of Allergy and Applied Immunology*, **18,** 348.
12. Gough, J. (1961) Post-mortem differences in asthma and chronic bronchitis. *Acta Allergologica*, **16,** 391.
13. Urschell, H. C., Paulson, D. L. and Shaw, R. R. (1966) Mucoid impaction of the bronchi. *American Thoracic Surgery*, **2,** 1.

14. Spencer, H. (1968) In *Pathology of the Lung*, 2nd edn. Oxford: Pergamon, 715, 720.
15. Szentivanyi, A. (1968) The beta adrenergic theory of atopic abnormality in bronchial asthma. *Journal of Allergy*, **42,** 203.
16. Lichtenstein, L. M. and Gillespie, E. (1973) Inhibition of histamine release by histamine controlled by H2 receptor. *Nature*, **244,** 287.
17. Parker, C. W., Huber, M. G. and Baumann, M. L. (1973) Alterations in cyclic AMP metabolism in human bronchial asthma. Journal of *Clinical Investigation*, **52,** 1342.
18. Parker, C. W. and Smith, J. W. (1973) Alerations in cyclic adenosine monophosphate metabolism in human bronchial asthma. *Journal of Clinical Investigation*, **52,** 48.
19. McFadden, E. R., Kiser, R., DeGroot, W. J. (1973) Acute bronchial asthma: Relations between clinical and physiologic manifestations. *New England Journal of Medicine*, **288,** 221.
20. Despas, P. J., Leroux, M. and Macklem, P. J. (1972) Site of airway obstruction in asthma as determined by measuring maximal expiratory flow breathing air and a helium-oxygen mixture. Journal of Clinical Investigation, **51,** 3235.
21. McCarthy, D. and Milic-Emili, J. (1973) Closing volume in asymptomatic asthma. *American Review of Respiratory Diseases*, **107,** 559.
22. Hill, D. J., Landau, L. I. and Phelan, P. D. (1972) Small airway disease in asymtomatic asthmatic adolescents. *American Review of Respiratory Diseases*, **106,** 873.
23. Tattersfield, A. E., Leaver, D. G. and Pride, N. B. (1973) Effects of B adrenergic blockade and stimulation on normal human airways. *Journal of Applied Physiology*, **35,** 613.
24. McNeill, R. S. and Ingram, C. G. (1966) Effect of propranolol on ventilatory function. *American Journal of Cardiology*, **18,** 473.
25. Sweatman, W. J. F. and Collier, H. O. J. (1968) Effects of prostaglandins on human bronchial muscle. *Nature*, **217,** 336.
26. Mathe, A. A. Hedquist, P., Holmgren, A. and Scanborg, N. (1973) Bronchial hyperreactivity to prostaglandin F_2 and histamine in patients with asthma. *British Medical Journal*, **1,** 193.

CHAPTER 4

The Immunology of Asthma

H. Amos

CHILDHOOD ASTHMA IS a manifestation of atopy and as such has genetic, immunological and pharmacological implications. The tissue damage resulting from an asthmatic attack has features in common with experimentally induced anaphylaxis. This condition is brought about by IgE-mediated release of histamine and other pharmacologically active substances which then exert a local effect on the surrounding target tissue, such as smooth muscle and blood vessels. A similar sequence of events may be involved in the pathogenesis of atopic asthma. Adult asthma is largely non-atopic and probably related to the deposition of antigen-antibody complexes with the subsequent fixation of complement.[1]

The findings from experimental models of anaphylaxis have been liberally applied to atopic asthma in an attempt to understand the disease. Any model, however, must explain the facts that are known to relate to the clinical syndrome. These are –

1. the pathological findings in the lungs during an acute attack;
2. a strong familial tendency to acquire the atopic condition;
3. an associated IgE antibody response to various allergens; and
4. the effectiveness of therapeutic agents that relax bronchial tone.

The essence of this chapter is to examine these facts to see if they are compatible with an immunologically induced disease state.

Pathology. As pointed out earlier, the striking features of the gross lung pathology following death in status asthmaticus are over-inflation and extensive plugging of the small 2 to 4 mm bronchi with viscid mucus. The presence of large numbers of eosinophils and the relative absence of neutrophils are features of an immunological phenomenon. The same cellular infiltration and over-inflated lungs are also found in animals dying from anaphylaxis.

Genetic aspects of atopic asthma. Much has been written about the precise definition of the term atopy and about the notion it was originally intended to convey. Most clinicians would agree that it is a useful term to describe a group of diseases that may occur together within an individual. Asthma, eczema and hay fever comprise the established triad but other allergic diseases may sometimes be included. This particular triad has a strong familial tendency which suggests that heredity may be an important aetiological factor. The evidence supporting an hereditary element for the atopic diseases as a group comes from two lines of study. Firstly, investigations into families have shown that the incidence of atopic disease is higher when the propositii are atopic than in families where there are non-atopic propositii.[24] Secondly, it was found that monozygotic twins have concordance in atopic disease more than discordance. In dizygotic twins the concordance is less marked.[5]

Pepys[1] uses the term atopy to mean 'the capacity to produce IgE as evidenced by skin test or serum IgE levels'. In the context of this definition hereditary factors are likely to be closely related to the ability to produce reaginic (IgE) antibody. Pertinent to the concept of atopy are the experiments of Levine and his colleagues,[6] who injected groups of mice from eight different inbred strains (A/He, CBA, C3H, AKR, C57B, C59L, SWR, SJL) with protein antigens and assayed the serum for reaginic and IgG_1 antibodies. They were able to demonstrate that a single large injection of antigen (100 μg) induced an antibody response in all eight strains but repeated injections of minute doses of antigen (0·1 μg) produced responses in only the A/He, CBA, C3H and AKR strains. Moreover, the low dose regime preferentially favoured reaginic antibody production which could still be detected up to twenty weeks after the initial injection. An extension of this work showed that the ability to respond to the antigen injections correlated with the H–2 genotype.[7,8] This finding with protein antigen is of considerable interest as it confirms the experiments of McDevitt and Chinitz[9] who showed that an H–2 linked locus controlled the immune response to injected synthetic antigens which have a more restricted antigenic heterogeneity.

McDevitt and his co-workers[10] termed this controlling locus the Ir–1 gene. It was shown subsequently, by genetic mapping, to be placed between the K end of the H–2 system and the SS–SLP locus.[11]

The conclusions drawn from the data obtained in the mouse system of Levine and colleagues has been considered a model for human atopy. Thus, atopy could be regarded as a genetically controlled ability to produce antibodies on repeated exposure to minute doses of antigen rather than as a unique ability to synthesise reagins.

More conclusive evidence for the existence of a genetically controlled immune response in atopic subjects is the demonstration of an antigen-specific Ir gene in human ragweed pollenosis. Levine, Stember and Fotino[12] analysed seven families in which ragweed hay fever occurred in more than one member and found that the association of HL–A haplotypes with IgE antibodies specific for the ragweed antigen (E) correlated with the hypersensitivity state. Such an association existing through successive generations of the seven families studied was interpreted as demonstrating a close genetic linkage between the HL-A system and a genetic locus controlling the immune response to antigen (E). By analogy with the mouse system it is likely that this is a demonstration of Ir gene expression.

Although these studies are of considerable importance, the inheritance of antigen-specific Ir genes is not sufficient to account for the atopic trait. Other inherited factors such as the permeability of mucus membranes and environmental factors are also of some importance.[13]

Hypersensitivity mechanisms in asthma

Allergens. Telling evidence for an immunological role in the aetiology of asthma is the association between asthmatic attacks and unusual environmental antigens like castor bean.[14] From these early observations of causal relationships more quantitative procedures have been sought which allow scientific analysis of the hypersensitivity state. Active material has been extracted from grass, trees, fur, feathers, mites and moulds, which, when injected into the skin of an asthmatic individual, may produce a wheel and flare reaction within 15 to 20 minutes of the injection.

The major problem associated with the preparation of allergens has been and still is, one of standardisation. The first attempt at obtaining uniform preparations was made by Noon,[15] who devised a unit based on weight of crude dried extract in relation to volume of extracting fluid. Noon was working on allergic rhinitis and the unit was therefore known as the pollen unit, equivalent to the amount of material extracted from 1 μg of pollen. When it became apparent that the active ingredient in the allergen extract was protein, a unit based on protein nitrogen was established.[16] Proteins were precipitated from crude extracts by phaphotungistic acid and the nitrogen in the precipitate determined by Kjeldahl analysis. The protein nitrogen unit (PNU) was set at l ng N. Most of the commercially produced allergen extracts currently available are calibrated in terms of the PNU but it is important to remember that standardising extracts by means of total protein nitrogen may bear little relation to the biological activity of the material. Various proteins in pollen are not antigenically active and the amount of actual antigen from the same species of grass may vary from year to year even though extraction procedures are the same.[17] Furthermore, the chemical manipulations used to prepare the extract may cause denaturation of proteins resulting in loss of activity without affecting the total nitrogen content. Thus, the PNU needs to be replaced by some measure of biological activity. Work is certainly progressing in this direction and many preparations are now being standardised by double layer gel diffusion against a standard allergen preparation.

Nature of the reagin. One of the most significant advances in understanding the pathogenesis of asthma was the indentification of the reaginic antibody. In 1966, Ishizaka, Ishizaka and Hornbrook[18] isolated a protein from the sera of asthmatic patients and showed that it had marked reaginic activity. The protein could not be related to any of the existing classes of immunoglobulins so a new class, designated IgE, was established. The concentration of IgE in the serum of healthy adults ranges from 0·1 to 0·7 μg per ml ($\pm$125 i.u./ml); this is extremely low compared with the concentrations of other serum immunoglobuins. From the discovery of IgE myeloma considerable information has accumulated on the physical and functional properties of the IgE molecule.[19] It has a molecular weight of 200,000 and sediments at 8·2. In common with IgG, papain digestion splits the molecule into two (Fab) fragments carrying the antibody combining sites and a crystalline piece (Fc). Both ends of the IgE antibody make an important contribution to its rather unique functional properties. It is the Fc end of the immunoglobulin that binds to mast cells and basophils and about 10,000 to 40,000 molecules become attached to each cell. This is the same for atopic and non-atopic subjects. As the antibody combining sites are not involved in cellular attachment they are free to combine with antigen and, if two or more IgE molecules are cross-linked by antigen, histamine is released from the cells. Histamine is also released if the cross-linking is effected by anti-IgE. The ease with which antigen combination can bring about histamine release is related to the number of IgE molecules on the sensitised cell. Ishizaka, Soto and Ishizaka[20] demonstrated convincingly that the figure 10,000 to 40,000 molecules per cell did not represent saturation of IgE receptor sites; more molecules were taken up if basophils from an allergised individual were incubated *in vitro* with IgE myeloma serum. The amount of IgE bound to the cells *in vivo* is therefore the result of an equilibrium reflecting the reversibility of the binding. This is important, as it has been shown that the more molecules there are attached to a cell the less anti-IgE is needed to effect maximum histamine release.[20]

Atopic diseases tend to be associated with raised serum IgE levels. About 50 per cent of patients with allergic asthma, for example, have markedly raised IgE levels.[21] The highest serum levels are found in those patients who are skin-test positive to multiple antigens and have been subjected to repeated antigen exposure. During the pollen season an asthmatic patient may have a very high level of serum IgE which reverts to normal during the winter. This finding is compatible with the short serum half-life of IgE and continued synthesis in the presence of antigen. Serum levels of IgE are comparatively easy to measure but they may be of little relevance to the intensity of the hypersensitivity state. This is because IgE has a very high affinity for tissue cells (association constant in the region of 109/mole) and remains attached to the cells during their lifespan. Thus, a patient may have a normal serum IgE level but still be capable of mounting a hypersensitivity reaction.

Attention has been directed recently towards a short-term sensitising IgG antibody in humans which can initiate the anaphylactic release of histamine.[22] Unlike IgE it is not destroyed by heating to 56°C for 6 hours and it will resist sulphydryl reduction. Although it binds to basophils, the association is weak compared with the high avidity of IgE. This short-term sensitising IgG antibody is probably not involved in the pathogenesis of childhood asthma. Its importance is probably in relation to asthma of late onset, which does not respond to treatment with sodium cromoglycate.

IgG precipitating antibodies may be responsible for producing a Type III allergic asthma[1] and clearly they must be distinguished from the IgG anaphylactic antibody. The mechanism by which they both produce tissue damage is quite distinct. In terms of the Coombs and Gell classification[23] anaphylactic antibodies produce damage by means of widespread release of pharmacologically active substances like histamine, while IgG precipitins produce a Type III damage mediated by antigen-antibody complexes and complement. Type III allergic asthma rarely if ever occurs in children. It is more relevant to adult asthma which develops independently of the atopic trait.

Target organ and target cells in allergic asthma. The organ primarily affected in an asthmatic attack is the lung but the tissue damage in the lung is secondary to an immunological reaction taking place on the surface of specific target cells. It has been clearly shown that reaginic antibody in several animal species will bind to a variety of cells. These include mast cells and basophils,[24,25] rat leucocytes,[26] and rabbit platelets.[27] There is general agreement that in most species, including humans, mast cells and/or basophils are the primary target cells in Type I allergic damage, but Tomioka and Ishizaka[28] showed that the mast cell is the only cell in primate lung to which IgE myeloma protein will bind.

The mast cell was known to be important in allergic asthma from the experiments of Salvato,[29] who demonstrated that fewer intact mast cells could be detected in the lungs during an acute asthmatic attack than in normal individuals. Mast cell debris, including granules, was also more readily observed in the connective tissue of the lungs during an attack. The distribution of mast cells within the lung is obviously of some relevance if the tissue damage results from IgE-induced degranulation. Brinkman[30] showed that the majority of mast cells were to be found randomly distributed in the submocosa; very few were demonstrated actually in the mucosa. By analysing brush biopsies, Patterson, Susko and Zeiss[31] were able to show primate mast cells free in the bronchial lumen, a site that would facilitate contact with inhaled allergens. This site is of some significance since Richardson and associates[32] found that antigen inhaled by an allergised animal did not penetrate further than the epithelial lining of the bronchi. Thus, the first stage in an asthmatic attack is probably allergen reacting with IgE-sensitised mast cells at the epithelial surface of the bronchi. Mast cells deep in the interstices of the lungs are probably not involved in the reaction.

Consequences of mast cell degranulation. Morphological studies on mast cells[30,33,34] have not revealed any unique features of the cells from atopic subjects. It is likely then that the abnormality in atopics is related to the antibody rather than to malformed target cells.

The effect of antigen combining with IgE antibody and cross-linking it on the surface of mast cells is to induce degranulation. This leads to the release of potent pharmacological mediators which are either stored in the cell like histamine or are synthesised like slow reacting substances of anaphylaxis (SRS–A) from precursor substances at the time of cell activation.

Histamine is the major pharmacological mediator stored in mast cells. In *in vitro* model systems it can be shown to constrict bronchial smooth muscle and it can be detected in asthmatic lungs after *in vitro* challenge with specific antigen.[35,36] Despite these findings it is doubtful whether histamine plays a significant role in causing the bronchospasm experienced by asthmatics.[37] In fact, recent work, particularly by Lichenstein and Bourne,[38] ascribes a role to histamine that is different from the straightforward expression of pharmacological activity. These workers found that histamine can activate adenyl cyclase, the enzyme that catalyses the formation of 3′ 5′ AMP from ATP,[39] which then effectively inhibits further production of the amine. Thus, histamine may control the magnitude of the response of sensitised tissues to antigen.

SRS–A is distinct from histamine in that it can contract smooth muscle in the presence of anti-histamine drugs.[36] Sheard and Blair[40] supported Brocklehurst's findings[36] by demonstrating that a perfusate from a passively sensitised human lung, when challenged with antigen, would contract a human bronchial strip, and that this contraction was due to SRS–A and not histamine. It is generally agreed that experiments of this type implicate SRS–A in the pathogenesis of atopic asthma, SRS–A acting directly on the bronchial smooth muscle.

A third substance released from mast cells is eosinophil chemotactic factor (ECF–A), a low molecular weight acid peptide which selectively attracts eosinophils into the area of release.[41] The full functional role of eosinophils in allergic asthma is at present unknown. The experiments of Orange and colleagues[42] would suggest that eosinophils secrete an enzyme, arylsulphatase, which can inhibit the action of SRS–A. If these experiments are confirmed, one effect of eosinophils could be to regulate the amount of free SRS–A.

Prostaglandins are long chain fatty acids which have a potent effect on smooth muscle and blood vessels.[43] The E series, PGE_1 and PGE_2 act as bronchodilators,[44] whereas PGF_2 is a bronchoconstrictor.[45] It is unlikely that prostaglandins are released as a primary consequence of antigenic challenge to passively sensitised mast cells but they do appear in the perfusate of lung fragments challenged with antigen.[46] It is thought, therefore, that they are synthesised as a result of the primary immunological reaction and then exert their effect on the bronchial smooth muscle. An important property of the prostaglandins is their effect on the cyclic nucleotide 3′ 5′ AMP. The E series tend to increase the level of cyclic AMP, thus inhibiting further production of histamine, while PGF_2 decreases the intercellular level of C–AMP stimulating histamine production.

Control of mediator expression. In most biological systems involving the mediators of homeostasis there are various feedback pathways which limit the extent of the response. The key to control Type I allergic tissue damage is 3′ 5′ AMP. Sutherland and Robinson[39] showed that adrenergic drugs react with receptors in tissues to activate adenyl cyclase and increase the level of C–AMP. Increasing the intracellular level of C–AMP effectively reduces the amount of histamine and SRS–A released from human fragments challenged with antigen.[42] It is now known that, in addition to the catecholamines, histamine itself and the E prostaglandins can all bring about an increase in C–AMP with subsequent switching off of further mediator production.[47,48] The experiments of Orange and colleagues[49] on the inhibition of SRS–A by eosinophil arylsulphatase shows that mechanisms also exist to control the action of mediators once they have been formed. The inactivation of C–AMP is brought about by the action of a second enzyme, phosphodiesterase, which can be inhibited by the methylxanthine drugs. Inhibition maintains the elevated intracellular level of C–AMP and prevents continued secretion of mediators. It is probable that this is the mechanism for the effectiveness of theophyllins in the treatment of asthmatics.

In view of the adrenergic stimulation of C–AMP it is not surprising there should be a cholinergic stimulus that enhances the antigen-induced release of histamine and SRS–A.[50,51] The experiments of Gold, Kessler and Yu,[52] demonstrating that atropine may block antigen-induced bronchospasm, suggest that cholinergic receptors may exist in human lung tissue. The cholinergic effect has been shown to be modulated in some tissues by the cyclic nucleotide guanosine 3′ 5′ monophosphate (C–GMP),[53,54] thus the two cyclic mucleotides may act in balance with one another to regulate the cellular function.

Speculation

Allergic asthma is a complicated multifactorial disease involving closely interwoven immunological and pharmacological mechanisms. Although the reaction sequence and control mechanisms of Type I allergic tissues damage, as typified by anaphylaxis, are gradually being elucidated, they do not fully explain the pathological findings in asthmatic lungs. At the present time no satisfactory explanation can be given for the increases in goblet cells and viscid mucus secretion which dominate the pathological picture.

Perhaps the effect of mediators on the afferent vagal nerve fibres, resulting in reflex bronchoconstriction and increased secretion, may be a more pertinent explanation of the findings.[51] Whatever the final mechanism may be, the immunologically-induced release of mediators is still likely to remain the most significant trigger for an asthmatic attack.

References

1. Pepys, J. (1973) Immunological mechanisms in asthma. Disodium cromoglycate. Proceedings ed. by J. Pepys and A. W. Frankland, Butterworths, London, 6.
2. Cooke R. A. and Vander Veer A. jr. (1916) Human Sensitisation. *Journal of Immunology*, **1,** 201.
3. Spain, W. C. and Cooke, R. A. (1924) Studies in specific hypersensitivity. II. The familial incidence of hay fever and bronchial asthma. *Journal of Immunology*, **9,** 521.
4. Adkinson, A. D. K. (1924) The behaviour of bronchial asthma as an inherited characteristic. *Genetics*, **5,** 363.
5. Spaich, D. and Ostertag, M. (1936) Zeitschrift für mensch; vererb und konstitutionsle hre. **19,** 731.
6. Levine, B. B. and Vaz, N. M. (1970) Effect of combinations of strain antigen dose and reagin producuion in the mouse. A model for human atopy. *International Archives of Allergy and Immunology*, **39,** 156.
7. Vaz, N. M. and Levine, B. B. (1970) Immune responsiveness of inhibited mice to known doses of antigen; relationship of histocompatibility (H–2) type. *Science*, **168,** 852.
8. Vaz, N. M., Phillips-Quagliata, J. M., Levine, B. B. and Vaz, E. M. (1971) H_2-linked genetic control of immune responsiveness to ovalbumin and ovomucoid. *Journal of Experimental Medicine*, **134,** 1335.
9. McDevitt, M. O., Chinitz, H (1969) Genetic control of antibody response relationship between immune response and histocompatibility, (H_2) type. *Science*, **163,** 1207.
10. McDevitt, M. O., Deak, B. D., Schreffler, D. C., Klein, J., Strimpfling, J. H., and Snell, G. D. (1972) Genetic control of the immune response. Mapping of the lr—1 locus. *Journal of Experimental Medicine*, **135,** 1529.

11. Luberman, R. A. and Humphrey, W. jr. (1972) Separation of Ir genes for IgG and IgA allotypes in mouse. *Federation Proceedings*, **31,** 777.
12. Levine, B. B., Stember, R. H. and Fotina, M. (1972) Ragweed hay fever: Genetic control and linkage of HL–A haplotypes. *Science*, **178,** 1201.
13. Salvaggio, J., Kayman, H. and Leskowitz, S. (1966) Immunologic responses in atopic and normal individuals to aerosolized dextran. *Journal of Allergy*, **38,** 31.
14. Figler, K. D. and Elrod, R. H. (1928) Endemic asthma due to castor bean dust. *Journal of the American Medical Association*, **90,** 79.
15. Noon, L. (1911) Prophylactic inoculation for hay fever. *Lancet*, 1572.
16. Cooke, R. A. and Stull, A. (1935) Preparation and standardisation of pollen extracts for the treatment of hay fever. *Journal of Experemental Medicine*, 62, 733.
17. Sherman, W. B. (1957) Reaginic and blocking antibodies. *Journal of Allergy*, **28,** 62.
18. Ishizaka, K., Ishizaka, T. and Hornbrook, M. N. (1966) Physico-chemical properties of reaginic antibody. IV. Presence of a unique immunoglobulin as a carrier of reaginic activity. *Journal of Immunology*, **97,** 75.
19. Johansson, S. G. O. and Bennich, H. (1967) Immunological studies of an atypical (myeloma) immunoglobulin. *Immunology*, **13,** 381.
20. Ischizaka, T. Soto, C. S. and Ishizaka, K., (1973) Mechanisms of passive sensitization. III Number of IgE molecules and their receptor sites on human basophil granulocytes. *Journal of Immunology*, **111,** 599.
21. Johansson, S. G. O., Foucard, T. and Dannaeus, A. (1974) IgE in human disease. In *Progress in Allergy II*, p. 61. (Ed. Brent, L and Holborow, J.) Amsterdam: North Holland Publishing Co.
22. Parish, W. E. (1970) Short term anaphylactic IgG antibodies in human sera. *Lancet*, **12,** 591.
23. Coombs, R. R. A. and Gell, P. G. H. (1953) *Clinical Aspects of Immunology*. Oxford: Blackwell, 575.
24. Mota, I. and Vugman, I. (1956) Effects of anaphylactic shock compound 48/80 on the mast cells of a guinea-pig lung. *Nature*, **177,** 427.
25. Orange, R. P., Stechshulte, D. and Austen, K. F. (1970) Immunochemical and biological properties of rat IgE. *Journal of Immunology*, **105,** 1087.
26. Orange, R. P., Valentine, M. D. and Austen, K. F. (1968) Antigen induced release of cell reacting substance of anaphylaxis (SRS–A) in rats prepared with homologous antibody. *Journal of Experimental Medicine*, **127,** 767.
27. Henson, P. M. and Cochrane, C. G. (1969) Immunological induction of increased vascular permeability: 1. A rabbit passive cutaneous anaphylactic reaction requiring complement platelets and neutrophils. *Journal of Experiemental Medicine*, **129,** 153.
28. Tomioka, H. and Ishizaka, K. (1971) Mechanisms of passive sensitisation. II Presence of receptors for IgE on monkey mast cells. *Journal of Immunology*, **107,** 971.
29. Salvato, G. (1961) Mast cells in bronchial connective tissue in man. *International Archives of Allergy and Immunology*, **18,** 348.
30. Brinkman, G. L. (1968) The mast cell in normal bronchus and lung. *Journal of Ultrastructure Research*, **23,** 115.
31. Patterson, R., Susko, I. M. and Zeiss, C. R. (1972) Reactions of primate respiratory mast cells. *Journal of Allergy and Clinical Immunology*, **50,** 7.
32. Richardson, J. B., Hogg, J. C., Bouchard, T. and Hall, D. L. (1973) Localisation of antigen in experimental bronchial constriction in guinea pig. *Journal of Allergy and Clinical Immunology*, **52,** 172.
33. Orr, T. S. C. (1973) Mast Cells and allergic asthma. *British Journal of Diseases of the Chest*, **67,** 1.
34. Weinstock, A. and Albright, J. T. (1967) The fine structure of mast cells in normal human gingiva. 17, 245. *Journal of Ultrastructure Research*, **17,** 245.
35. Schild, H. O., Haskins, D. F., Mongar, J. L. and Hexrxheimer, H. (1951) Reactions of isolated human asthmatic lung on bronchial tissue of a specific antigen. *Lancet*, **2,** 376.
36. Brocklehurst, W. E. (1960) The release of histamine and the formation of a slow reacting substance (SRS–A) during anaphylactic shock. *Journal of Physiology*, **15,** 416.

37. Austen, K. F. and Blannerhasset, J. (1968) Bronchial asthma. In *Textbook of Immunopathology*, p. 256 (Ed. Meischer P. A. and Muller-Eberhard H. J.) New York: Grune and Stratton.
38. Lichtenstein, L. M. and Bourne, H. R. (1971) Inhibition of allergic histamine release by histamine and other agents which stimulate adenyl cyclase. In *Biochemistry of the Acute Allergic Reactions.* (Ed. Austen K. F. and Becker E. L.) Oxford: Blackwell.
39. Sutherland, E. W. and Robinson, G. A. (1966) The role of cyclic 3′ 5′ AMP in responses to catecholamines and other hormones. *Pharmacological Reviews*, **18,** 145.
40. Sheard, P. and Blair, A. M. J. N. (1970) Disodium cromoglycate activity in three *in vitro* models of immediate hypersensitivity reaction in lung. *International Archives of Allergy and Immunology*, **38,** 217.
41. Kay, A. B. and Austen, K. F. (1971) The IgE-mediated release of an eosinophil leukocyte chemotactic factor from human lung. *Journal of Immunology*, **107,** 899.
42. Orange, R. P., Austen, W. G. and Austen, K. F. (1971) The immunological release of histamine and cell reacting substances of anaphylaxis from human lung. 1. Modulation by agents influencing cellular levels of cyclic 3′ 5′ adenosine monophosphate. *Journal of Experimental Medicine*. **134,** 1365.
43. Horton, E. V. (1956) Biological activities of pure prostaglandins. *Experientia (Basel)*, **21,** 113.
44. Cuthbert, M. F. (1969) The effect on airways resistance of prostaglandins E, administered by aerosol to healthy and asthmatic volunteers. *British Medical Journal*, **4,** 723.
45. Swetman, W. J. F. and Collier, H. O. J. (1968) Effect of prostaglandins on human bronchial muscle. *Nature*, **217,** 69.
46. Piper, P. J. and Walker, J. L. (1973) The release of spasmogenic substances from human chopped lung tissue and its inhibition. *British Journal of Pharmacology*, **47,** 291.
47. Bourne, H. R., Melmon, K. L. and Lichtenstein, L. M. (1971) Histamine augments leukocyte adenosine 3′ 5′ monophosphate and blocks antigenic histamine release. *Science*, **173,** 743.
48. Bourne, H. R. and Lichternstein, L. M. and Melmon, K. (1972) Pharmacologic control of allergic histamine release *in vitro*: evidence for an inhibitory role of 3′ 5′ adenosine monophosphate in human leukocytes. *Journal of Immunology*, **108,** 695.
49. Orange, R., Murphy, R. C. and Austen, K. F. (1974) Inactivation of slow reacting substances of anaphylaxis (SRS–A) by arylsulfatases. *Journal of Immunology*, **113,** 316.
50. Kaliner, M., Orange, R. P. and Austen, K. F. (1972) Immunological release of histamine and slow reacting substances of anaphylaxis from human lung. IV. Enhancement of cholinergic and adrenergic stimulation. *Journal of Experimental Medicine*, **136,** 556.
51. Orange R. P. (1973) Immunopharmacological aspects of bronchial asthma. *Clinical Allergy*, **3,** 521.
52. Gold, W. M., Kessler, G. and Yu, D. Y. C. (1973) Vagally mediated reflex bronchoconstriction in allergic asthma. 16th Aspen Europhysema Conference, Aspen, Colorado (in press).
53. George, W. J., Polson, J. F., O'Toole, A. G. and Goldberg, N. D. (1970) Elevation of guanosine 3′ 5′ cyclic phosphate in rat heart after perfusion with acylcholine. *Proceedings of the National Academy of Sciences*, **66,** 398.
54. Kuo, J., Lee, T., Reyes, P. L., Walton, K. F., Donnelly, T. E. and Greengard, P. (1972) Cyclic neucleotide-dependent protein kinases. An assay method for the measurement of guanosine 3′ 5′ monophosphate on various biological materials and a study of agents reacting dose level in heart and brain. *Journal of Biological Chemistry*, **247,** 16.

CHAPTER 5

Lung Function Tests and Their Interpretation

Jan A. Kuzemko and S. Bedford

IN RELATION TO adults, children have small lungs, and the respiratory muscles are in the process of development. Thus, any test of lung function will not only be influenced by the age and stature of the child but also by his active co-operation. In general, the child of 6 years and over can be assessed fully and adequately; the child of 3 to 6 years can often co-operate in using a Wright's Peak Flow meter (low range model). With the exception of infants[1,2] there are no satisfactory lung function tests for children aged 1 to 3 years, but a special adaptation of the body plethysmography is being developed.[3] Total body plethysmography is really a research tool and because of its cost and maintenance, it is doubtful if it will ever be widely used.

Lung function tests are best related to the child's body size rather than to his age since children of similar ages commonly vary in size. An isolated test or tests performed at random are of little clinical value. Whatever lung function tests are performed in children, there exist wide variations in normal values—on average $\pm$15 per cent about the mean. Thus, it is of utmost importance to calibrate one's equipment periodically, determine one's own laboratory normal values especially for BTPS (body temperature and pressure with 100 per cent water vapour saturation) and utilise several different tests to assess lung function. An excellent critical review of techniques and normal values has been compiled by Polgar and Promadhat.[4]

Methods

Lung volumes—
- Tidal Volume (TV)
- Expiratory Reserve Volume (ERV)
- Residual Volume (RV)

Vital Capacity (VC)
Functional Residual Capacity (FRC)
Total Lung Capacity (TLC)

Pappenheimer[5] and colleagues established a standard of symbols and definitions currently used in respiratory physiology. Lung volumes have two divisions: the volumes of air the child can breathe are called dynamic volumes, and the volume of air left in the lung at the end of voluntary expiration is termed Functional Residual Capacity (FRC). Normal respiration at rest is called Tidal Volume (TV). Vital Capacity (VC) is the maximum expulsion of air from the lungs following a maximum inspiration. The total volume of air present in the lungs is termed Total Lung Capacity (TLC). The Residual Volume (RV) is the volume of air left in the lungs at the end of forced expiration and the Expiratory Reserve Volume (ERV) is the maximal volume of gas that can be expired from the end—expiratory level. (Fig. 5.1)

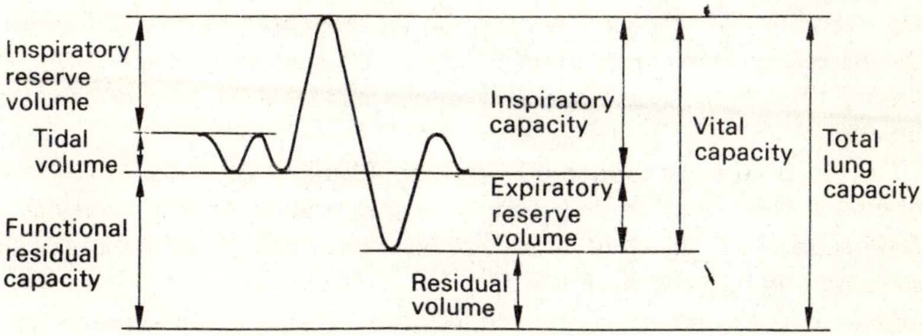

Fig. 5.1

These measurements can easily be made with any type of spirometer. In our experience, children aged six years have no difficulty in using a 9 litre Bell Capacity Spirometer, and many younger children, especially boys, prefer using an electronic spirometer which does not provide a record of tracing but Vital Capacity, Forced Expiratory Volume in the first second (FEV_1), and Peak Expiratory Flow Rate (PEFR) are displayed digitally on this instrument. It is a useful apparatus but care should be taken since errors of measurement are easy to make. It is helpful to have a one-way valve so that the child's mouth can be in place from the beginning of inspiration.

Frequent assessment of Vital Capacity in the child with asthma is a useful measurement of pulmonary function since the test depends on the elasticity of the lungs and the chest muscles. Vital Capacity will be reduced in those children with asthma who have any degree of airway obstruction. Mean values for British children have been compiled by Lunn.[6]

The Timed Vital Capacity or, as is generally accepted, the Forced Expiratory Volume qualified by time interval (FEV_T) measures that part of vital capacity that is related to the time required to perform the measurement.[17] The test is much more reliable than total VC since it is the amount of air per unit of time that is measured. Thus, the volume of air exhaled can be measured during the first second or first two or three seconds. The first second volume correlates best with other tests of lung function and with clinical symptoms of asthma.[18]

Measurements of selected segments of the Vital Capacity led to the development of the Maximum Midexpiratory Flow (MMF)[19] and Maximal Expiratory Flow Rate (MEFR).[20] A number of simple, reliable and portable instruments that quantitatively measure 'the expiratory push' are now available. The best known is the Wright's Peak Flow Meter,[21] which works on the principle of a variable area orifice meter. A ratchet is attached to the vane so that only maximum flow rates are recorded. Values obtained are comparable to those obtained by pneumotachography, and there is little variation with repeated tests[6] provided these are properly performed. The instrument is available in two ranges: 60 to 1,000 litre/m and 20 to 200 litre/m. The lower range model is well tolerated by children of three years and over.

To perform the test properly the child should blow as *hard* as he can into the device. It is important to have a number of trial blows first and in cases of difficulty to ask the child initially to blow out a candle and then blow in the same way into the meter.

As with all equipment, frequent checks are necessary as wide variations have been found between any two meters, sometimes as much as 15 per cent.

The Functional Residual Capacity (FRC) is a specialised test that can be performed in most children over six years of age and the results are reproducible to about 4 per cent. There are three techniques—

(*a*) A closed circuit helium dilution method.[7]
(*b*) An open circuit nitrogen washout method.[8]
(*c*) A total body plethysmography[9] which will also provide means of measuring airway resistance (airway resistance = alveolar pressure/air flow).

For details of methods and interpretation of results the reader is referred to the standard work of Cotes[11] and others.[12–14]

Measurement of FRC is of value diagnostically in children with asthma who develop only a minimal bronchoconstriction on exercise testing and, in remission, when it can be shown that FRC is increased and persists for many days following even a mild attack of asthma despite the fact that clinically the lungs appear normal.[15,38] More recently, Palmer and Kelman,[16] studying 35 adults, showed that although there was no obvious evidence of significant airways obstruction as demonstrated by simple spirometry, all patients had pulmonary hyperinflation, arterial hypoxaemia and hypocapnia when tested with specialised and sensitive techniques.

Exercise as diagnostic test

The lability index. A rational physiological classification of asthma in childhood has been developed by Jones.[21] The FEV_1 was measured with the child at rest. Following an exercise period of eight minutes, FEV_1 was re-measured in terms of its fall below the value at rest. After a return to the resting level, maximum bronchial dilatation was obtained by giving isoprenaline aerosol followed by a very brisk exercise of two minutes duration. The difference between the highest and lowest values for FEV_1 were expressed as a percentage of the predicted normal. Thus—

$$\text{Lability Index} = \frac{\text{Fall of } FEV_1 + \text{Rise of } FEV_1}{{}^{*}\,\text{Predicted normal } FEV_1} \times 100$$

*(In the normal child FEV_1 at rest replaces the predicted normal FEV_1.

Using this technique, Jones was able to divide asthmatic children into three groups—

	Lability Index
Group I	15–30%
Group II	>30%
Group III	Variable, FEV_1 at rest↓
Normal	< 20%

In general, Group I children are those suffering from mild clinical asthma with infrequent attacks; Group II children have moderate symptoms, are often atopic, and respond very well to sodium cromoglycate. Group III children are those who have a fixed component (muscle hypertrophy and/or oedema, etc.) of the airway resistance sufficient to prevent bronchial dilatation to within normal limits, even at rest (severe asthma). The Group I children labile component (muscle spasm) is small but in Group II children it is large. With age, the labile component of the airway resistance has a tendency to decrease, especially after adolescence, and may even return to normal in some individuals. In some further studies it was shown that the labile component may still operate although the subject has ceased to have attacks of asthma.[22] Presumably, the individual may develop asthma in middle age, but longitudinal studies are not available to support or refute this view. A child who demonstrates a fixed component will most likely have it as an adult although his Lability Index may regress to Group II or even, in some cases, Group I. In all, over 80 per cent of children with asthma fall into Groups I and II. A child with a Lability Index of less than 15 per cent does not as a rule have asthma but some other reason for his symptoms. A method[1] based on these observations but utilising peak expiratory flow rates (PEFR) was described by Connolly and Godfrey.[23] Silverman and colleagues[24] studying various exercise tests found that the maximum degree of bronchoconstriction in a child with possible asthma was obtained by running on a treadmill six to eight minutes at about 5 km/hour with a slope of 10 to 15 per cent.

Types of exercise. There is a conflict of opinion as to the incidence of bronchoconstriction, mainly because of different methods of exercising and the use of different indices of testing respiratory function. Free running is undoubtedly the best bronchoconstrictor.[24,25] Swimming and walking have a small and variable effect.[26] Jones[21] states that practically all children develop exercise-induced bronchoconstriction, whereas Silverman and colleagues[24] (not using exactly the same exercise as Jones) found it in 73 per cent of children following a single test; when the negative responders were reassessed, the proportion of positive results increased to 95 per cent.[31] In a group of 100 consecutive children with asthma, we found the incidence of exercise-induced bronchoconstriction in 97 per cent. It is to be remembered that bronchoconstriction occurs after the exercise is completed, usually becoming maximal between four to six minutes.

An increased exercise lability has been observed in children who have had 'wheezy bronchitis', were symptom-free, and have not had clinical asthma.[27] In addition, near members of the family of asthmatic children who have themselves not suffered from asthma often have raised exercise lability.[28] Finally, in 50 per cent of children with cystic fibrosis, similar observations were made[29,39] although these results need confirmation.[40]

Precautions in carrying out exercise tests. In performing Exercise Tests in children, note should be taken of their clinical state during the preceding twenty four hours, and any possible treatment that may have been given inadvertently. There should be no hesitation in terminating the exercise if the child becomes breathless. In our experience, drugs are rarely needed to control exercise-induced bronchoconstriction. We believe that exercise testing should be done by the doctor himself as it is part of the total examination and assessment.

Needless to say, a single doubtful assessment should be repeated, and the Lability Index of Jones should be assessed periodically. In a series of 300 children during seven years, we have not so far found one instance of a false positive; 9 children who were suspected of having 'asthma', and had Lability Indices of less than 15 per cent, have remained well during five years of observation. For a comprehensive review of exercise testing in children, the reader should consult the publication of Godfrey,[30] or proceedings of a Symposium on Exercise and Asthma.[41]

Exercise-induced bronchoconstriction (EIB) and drug therapy. Sympathomimetic agents such as salbutamol, terbutaline, adrenaline and others inhibit EIB if administered before the exercise and modify EIB if given shortly after it.[32,33] Similarly, sodium cromoglycate can abolish EIB completely in a high proportion of children[34] when inhaled about 20 to 30 minutes before an average exercise or when given immediately before a very short exercise, e.g. five minutes. Corticosteroids,[35] inhaled steroids[36,37] and antihistamine drugs[35] have no effects on EIB.

Thus, a standard exercise test is most useful in those children whose symptoms occur predominantly following play and interfere with their normal activities. The effects, duration of action, possible side-effects of bronchodilators or other drugs can be studied, and rational advice to the child and his family offered.

References

1. Nelson, N. M. (1966) Neonatal pulmonary function. *Pediatric Clinics of N. America*, **13,** 3, 769.
2. Krieger, I (1963) Studies in mechanics of respiration in infancy. *American Journal of Diseases of Childhood*, **105,** 439.
3. Milner, A. D. (1970) The respiratory jacket. *Lancet*, **2,** 80.
4. Polgar, G. and Promadhat, V. (1971) Techniques and Standards for Pulmonary Function Tests in Children. Philadelphia: W. B. Saunders Co.
5. Pappenheimer, J. (1950) Standardisation of definitions and symbols in respiratory physiology. *Federation Proceedings*, **9,** 602.
6. Lunn, J. E. (1965) Respiratory measurements of 3556 Sheffield school children. *British Journal of Preventive and Social Medicine*, **19,** 115.
7. Gibson, J. C. and Hugh-Jones, P. (1949) The measurement of the total lung volume and breathing capacity. *Clinical Science*, **7,** 185.
8. Darling, R. C., Cournand, A. and Richards, D. W. (1940) Studies of intrapulmonary mixing gases.' *Journal of Clinical Investigation*, **19,** 609.
9. Dubois, A. B., Botelho, S. Y., Bedell, G. N., Marshall, R. and Comroe J. H. (1956) A rapid plethysmographic method of measuring thoracic gas volume: A comparison with a nitrogen washout method for measuring functional residual capacity in normal subjects. *Journal of Clinical Investigation*, **35,** 322.
10. Dubois, A. B., Botelho, S. Y. and Comroe, J. H. (1956) A new method for measuring airway resistance in man using a body plethysmograph: values in normal subjects and in patients with respiratory disease. *Journal of Clinical Investigation*, **35,** 327.
11. Cotes J. E. (1968) *Lung Function: Assessment and Application in Medicine*, 2nd edn. Oxford: Blackwell.
12. Engstrom, I., Karlberg, P. and Kraepelien, S. (1956) Respiratory studies in children. I. Lung volumes in healthy children 6–14 years of age. *Paediatrica Scandinavica*, **45,** 277.
13. Engstrom, I., Escardo, F. E., Karlberg, P. and Kraepelien, S. (1959) Respiratory studies in children VI. Timed vital capacity in healthy children and in symptom free asthmatic children. *Acta Paediatrica Scandinavica Supp.* 114.
14. Helliesen, P. J., Cook, C. D., Friedlander, L. and Agathon, S. (1958) Studies of

respiratory physiology in children I. Mechanics of respiration and lung volumes in 85 normal children 5–17 years of age. *Pediatrics*, **22,** 80.

15. Engstrom, I. (1964) Respiratory studies in children. XI. Mechanics of breathing lung volumes and ventilatory capacity in asthmatic children from attack to symptom free status. *Acta Paediatrica Scandinavica. Supp.* 155.
16. Palmer, K. N. V. and Kelman, G. R. (1975) Pulmonary function in asthmatic patients in remission. *British Medical Journal*, **1,** 485.
17. Gaensler, E. A. (1951) Analysis of the ventilation defect by times capacity measurements. *American Review of Tuberculosis and Pulmonary Disease*, **64,** 256.
18. Gandevia, B. and Hugh-Jones, P. (1957) Terminology for measurements of ventilatory capacity: A report to the Thoracic Society. *Thorax*, **12,** 290.
19. Leuallen, E. C. and Fowler, W. S. (1955) Maximal Midexpiratory Flow. *American Review of Tuberculosis and Pulmonary Disease*, **72,** 783.
20. Cander, L. and Comroe, J. H. (1955) A method for objective evaluation of bronchodilator drugs. *Journal of Allergy*, **26,** 210.
21. Wright, B. M. and McKerrow, C. B. (1959) Maximum forced expiratory flow rate as a measure of ventilatory capacity. *British Medical Journal*, **2,** 1041.
22. Blackhall, M.I. (1970) Ventilatory function in subjects with childhood asthma who have become symptom free. *Archives of Disease in Childhood*, **45,** 363.
23. Connolly, N. and Godfrey, S. (1970) Assessment of the child with asthma. *Journal of Asthma Research*, **8.** 31.
24. Silverman, M. and Anderson, S. D. (1972) Standardisation of Exercise Tests in Asthmatic Children. *Archives of Disease in Childhood*, **47,** 882.
25. Anderson, S. D., Connolly, N. M. and Godfrey, S. (1971) Comparison of bronchoconstriction induced by cycling and running. *Thorax*, **26,** 396.
26. Godfrey, S., Silverman, M. and Anderson, S.D. (1973) Problems of interpreting exercise-induced asthma. *Journal of Allergy and Immunology*, **52,** 4, 199.
27. Koñig, P., Godfrey, S. and Abrahamov, A. (1972) Exercise-induced bronchial lability in children with a history of wheezy bronchitis. *Archives of Disease in Childhood*, **47,** 458.
28. König, P. and Godfrey, S. (1973) Prevalence of exercise-induced bronchial lability in families of children with asthma. *Archives of Disease in Childhood*, **48,** 513.
29. Day, G. and Mearns, M. B. (1973) Bronchial Lability in Cystic Fibrosis. *Archives of Disease in Childhood*, **48,** 355.
30. Godfrey, S. (1974) *Exercise Testing in Children.* New York and London: W. B. Saunders.
31. Anderson, S. D., Silverman, M., König, P. and Godfrey, S. (1975) Exercise-induced asthma. *British Journal of Diseases of the Chest*, **69,** 1.
32. Jones, R. S., Wharton, M. J. and Buston, N. H. (1963) Place of physical exercise and bronchodilator drugs in the assessment of the asthmatic child. *Archives of Disease in Childhood*, **38,** 972.
33. Anderson, S. D., Dolton, R., Lindsay, D. A. and Rozea, P. (1974) Exercise challenge testing in asthmatic subjects—its usefulness in drug evaluation. *Australian and New Zealand Journal of Medicine*, **4,** 312.
34. Silverman, M., König, P. and Godfrey, S. (1973) The use of serial exercise tests to assess the efficiency and duration of action of drugs for asthma. *Thorax*, **28,** 574.
35. McNeill, R. S., Nairn, J. R., Miller, J. S. and Ingram, C. G. (1966) Exercise-induced asthma. *Australian Journal of Medicine*, **35,** 55.
36. Konig, P., Jaffe, P. J., and Godfrey, S. (1974) The effect of corticosteroids on exercise-induced asthma. *Journal of Allergy and Clinical Immunology*, **54,** 14.
37. Kuzemko, J. A. (Unpublished data)
39. McFadden, E. R. and Lyons, H. A. (1969) Serial studies of factors influencing airway dynamics during recovery from acute asthma attacks. *Journal of Applied Physiology*, **27,** 452.
39. Counahan, R. and Mearns, M. B. (1975) Prevalence of atopy and exercise-induced bronchial lability in relatives of patients with cystic fibrosis. *Archives of Disease in Childhood*, **50,** 477.

40. Jones, R. S. (1975) Bronchial lability in cystic fibrosis. *Archives of Disease in Childhood*, **11,** 909.
41. Symposium on Exercise and Asthma (1975) *Pediatrics* (Suppl.), **56,** 5, 843.

CHAPTER 6

History, Examination and Investigations

S. Bedford

Successful management of the asthmatic child presupposes adequate knowledge and understanding of both the child and his illness. As with all clinical problems, it is helpful to adopt a standardised approach that is flexible enough to take account of individual variability. The most important step is a full and detailed history.[1]

History

It is essential to learn from the parent the major symptoms of the child's illness, at first without direct questioning. The presenting symptoms commonly consist of recurrent cough, wheezing, breathlessness on exertion, fatigue, nocturnal, cough, long-standing bronchitis, nasal stuffiness and hay fever.

Triggering factors such as playing on grass, riding or tending a pony, playing with household pets such as dogs, cats, rabbits, hamsters and guinea-pigs, or birds such as canaries and budgerigars, are suggestive of allergy.

Certain weather conditions such as cold winds or, conversely, humid and oppressive days are sometimes spoken of as precipitating factors.

Emotional factors, such as examinations, visits to the cinema or the theatre or hospital, attending a party, laughing too heartily, chastisement, or scolding by a parent are other frequently associated events. Sometimes foods may be incriminated, e.g. milk products, eggs, nuts, chocolate, fish, or drugs such as aspirin.

The mother may associate the child's illness with recurrent respiratory infections, with various dusts, tobacco smoke and other inhalational irritants within the home environment, especially dampness and inefficient ventilation.

Direct questioning must next be used to determine, if possible, both true and false relationships between the symptoms and suggested causes, and this requires systematising the factors involved.

Many of the presenting symptoms suggest that allergy plays an important role in producing the illness. This must be brought out by questions concerning the child's environment, with particular reference to the bedroom, where the presence of animal and vegetable fibres in bedclothes, floor and window coverings, e.g. wool, cotton, kapok, feathers in pillows and eiderdowns, may be important vectors. A family history of allergic illness such as asthma, hay fever, urticaria, and eczema in near relations, would be helpful in diagnosing the atopic state.

Often a link can be found between *infection* and illness; for example upper respiratory infections (sore throat, nasal discharge and obstruction, otitis media, etc.).

Detailed questions concerning the child's *exercise-tolerance* are needed to find his response to various forms of exertion such as physical education in school, cross-country runs, games, swimming and ordinary play.

Careful and tactful questions designed to discover the *psychological* home background are needed, as emotional disturbances are often quoted as precipitating attacks of illness. Examples are broken homes, single-parent situations, unhappy interparental relationships and unhappy relationships between the child and his parents, the number of children in the family, and the child's birth ranking.

During questioning, an effort should be made to try to discover whether the illness has consisted of a single event or is one of a series and whether it is seasonal or perennial; and to establish the child's age at the first attack, the interval between attacks, their severity and duration, and whether the child is normal between attacks. If the patient is of school age it is helpful to know how much time is lost from school because of his illness. Are the incidents more common in the daytime or at night? What measures have been used to produce relief, and their efficacy? Has the child had hospital admissions for his attacks, and if so, how many? The replies to these questions may give a clear picture of the severity of the illness and the degree of limitation of the child's normal activities.

Lastly, it is useful to learn the child's early history, including details of the pregnancy, labour, birth weight, neonatal and early infantile progress. It is also necessary to establish whether he has had eczema or repeated respiratory infections, especially bronchiolitis.

Clinical Examination

A child should always be examined fully and undressed. On inspection, the behaviour of child and parent both individually and towards each other should be noted in order to establish a psychological base-line. The child may lean very much on the mother, who may react by either acceptance or rejection, by calmness or over-reaction. The mother's attitude towards her child's activities in the consulting room can be very illuminating. While the child may be quiet and inactive, especially during periods of respiratory difficulty, he may, conversely, be hyperactive and full of bravado.

At the first interview, the patient may be anxious and apprehensive, which may produce a lack of co-operation. This is most frequently seen where there is a long history of respiratory embarrassment, and when the parents are either over-protective or, on the other hand, unsympathetic.

Children with a long history of severe asthma often exhibit hunching of the shoulders and an appearance of short neck. Their faces often suggest nasal obstruction, which may be the result of adenoidal enlargement or intranasal mucosal thickening, with or without nasal discharge. A cushingoid appearance, with 'mooning' of the face, may be present if there has been long-term treatment with corticosteroid drugs or corticotrophins. There may be chest deformity, e.g. pigeon-breast, barrel chest or Harrison's sulcus. Other signs such as finger-clubbing or cyanosis may be present.

The *cardiovascular system.* A routine examination should be made and should include measurement of the brachial blood pressure, especially if there has been long-term treatment with corticosteroids. The presence of pulsus paradoxus may be an important sign of acute illness.[2]

The *respiratory system.* During remission, there may be no signs of abnormality. However, when the child is ill there may be subcostal and intercostal recession, limitation of respiratory excursion, and over-use of the accessory muscles of respiration. Percussion may reveal hyperresonance if the lungs are hyperinflated or impairment of resonance in the presence of collapse and consolidation. *Auscultation* may reveal no abnormality during well periods. If, however, the child is ill, there may be limitation of air movement; the expiratory phase may be prolonged when the lungs are overinflated and the breath sounds may be bronchial or tubular in the presence of collapse-consolidation, which may be widespread or localised. Adventitious sounds such as rhonchi, expecially if expiratory and high-pitched, imply a degree of bronchial obstruction, while the presence of moist sounds such as râles and crepitations point to a probable infection. These latter signs may be widespread, lobar, or localised to smaller areas. Recurrent collapse-consolidation of the right middle lobe or lingula is sometimes the first and only feature of asthma in the young child.

The *ears* should be examined for evidence of past or present otitis media and hearing should be assessed broadly by whisper and watch-tick. Impairment of hearing and middle-ear damage may indicate the presence of enlargement and/or infection of adenoids.

The *nose.* Few doctors examine children's noses routinely. Yet, not uncommonly, the nose provides valuable clues to the diagnosis. In its anterior half, it is easily examined without recourse to mirror and speculum simply by raising the tip of the nose with one thumb and shining a light into the nasal cavity. It is quite easy to see the septum, the state of the nasal mucous membrane and also the middle and inferior turbinates. One should assess the patency of the nasal airways and the presence or absence of swelling of the mucosa. In the child with an allergic illness the mucosa will usually be swollen, pale and hypersecretive, while the turbinates are also swollen, often causing very marked obstruction. Occasionally, there may be nasal polypi which suggest the presence of chronic ethmoid sinusitis.[3] They are rare in children with asthma, although commoner in cystic fibrosis.[4] They may occur in a familial form and are sometimes associated with aspirin-sensitivity.[5]

The *pharynx*. In the pharynx, the tonsils are often small in some asthmatic children.[6] However, they may be enlarged, even grossly, and they may be inflamed and show irregularity and pitting of the surfaces, and there is frequently concommitant enlargement of the cervical lymph nodes. This is strongly suggestive of past infections, even if there is no evidence of active inflammation.

The *abdomen* should be examined routinely, as also the axillary and inguinal lymph nodes.

The *skin* must be examined for evidence of eczema, its extent, activity and severity, and the presence or absence of concommitant infection. In addition, there may be atrophic changes or even telangiectasia if topical applications of fluorinated corticosteroid preparations have been used for any length of time, especially on the face. The eczematous eruption is most commonly found in the flexures of elbows and knees, behind the ears, around the mouth and on the front of the trunk. The most severe lesions are often seen on the wrists, ankles, fingers and toes which may show painful fissuring.

Aids to Diagnosis

Chest radiography is mandatory as a routine investigation at the first attendance. While there is no 'typical' asthmatic X-ray picture, and nearly threequarters of asthmatic children show a normal pattern,[7] there may be abnormalities such as over-inflation, with a thin vertical heart and long narrow lungs with enlarged hilar vessels. The most marked signs occur in the most severe cases of constant asthma.

Routine radiography may show the presence of lobar or segmental collapse as the reason for absent air entry or unresolved pneumonia which may have been masked by increased wheeziness and dyspnoea. In addition, this may be the only way of revealing an inhaled foreign body.

Some children have asthmatic symptoms as a result of allergic broncho-pulmonary aspergillosis, which produces a characteristic radiological appearance.[7]

X-ray of the paranasal sinuses frequently shows opacity due to swelling of the mucous membrane in an allergic patient.

The wrist should be X-rayed to establish skeletal maturity, which, in conjunction with the child's height and weight and his chronological age, will establish a base-line on which to chart his growth pattern during the follow-up period.

The eosinophil leucocyte. This cell is a common denominator of many anaphylactic reactions which, generally, are associated with eosinophilia in peripheral blood.[8] The cells are believed to be attracted by antigen-antibody complexes and may be found in the lesions produced by anaphylactic reaction, e.g. the weal of urticaria.

Examination of the sputum and nasal secretions for the presence of eosinophils is easily carried out, and may add to the evidence supporting an allergic illness.[9] Also, a routine examination of the blood for haemoglobin, white cell count and total eosinophil count should be carried out.

It is important to note that accumulation of eosinophils in the periphery can be inhibited by antihistamines.

Relationship between asthma and hypersensitivity. The majority of asthmatic children are atopic, i.e. their illness appears to be related to allergy,[10] they tend to suffer from other types of allergic illness, (e.g. eczema, allergic rhinitis, hay fever) and there is a history of various allergic illnesses in near members of the family. One of the characteristics of the atopic individual is his ability to become sensitised easily to common allergens and thus develop multiple allergies. This type of hypersensitivity was termed Type I (anaphylactic) or Reagin-dependent by Gell and Coombes,[11] and it is mediated by a reaginic antibody, isolated by Ishizaka and colleagues, which has been labelled IgE.[12]

IgE is normally present in serum in small amounts—125 i.u./ml (0·03mg/100ml). It has the capacity of binding to mast cells and basophils which respond on further challenge with antigens by degranulation, with the release of histamine and other vasoactive amines. It is this release of active substances that appears to play a very important part in producing symptoms, e.g. broncho-constriction.

It would seem that IgE is not the only immunoglobulin responsible for immediate (Type I) allergic reactions, and that some may be due to short-term anaphylactic IgG antibodies.[13,14] Furthermore, immunological factors represent only part of the total picture of asthma and do not explain some important symptoms such as exercise-induced bronchoconstriction, and the response to emotional disturbance. Nor does Type I hypersensitivity explain the benefit of corticosteroids, which suppress Type III (Arthus) reactions, but do not inhibit Type I reactions.

However, as the child's history frequently points to a direct relationship between his illness and allergy, it is important to try to identify the substances to which he has become sensitised. The investigations in most common use for this purpose are—

skin sensitivity tests;
nasal and bronchial provocation tests;
radio-allergosorbent test (RAST);
identification of specific precipitating antibodies.

It is important that all sensitivity tests in children with seasonal illness should be carried out 'out of season', e.g. pollen asthma cases should be tested in November in England.[9]

Investigations

Skin Sensitivity Tests

These tests measure the response of the skin to challenge by various antigens. They need not necessarily be related to the response of bronchial mucosa, nor need they be related to the mechanism producing the actual illness.

For these reasons many workers consider that skin sensitivity tests are of limited value in the investigation of asthma[10,15] except in pollen related cases.[10] However, other workers consider that, if carried out correctly, related to the history, and combined with other tests such as RAST, they can give a very reliable picture.[16] Support may be sought from the effect of therapy by hyposensitisation and other methods.

The response of the skin (and other target organs) can be suppressed by antihistamine drugs, and they should therefore be withheld for the 24 to 48 hours preceding the tests.

The test almost universally in use is the prick-test. The intradermal test has been found to be too unreliable, tending to produce false positive results.

The test solutions should be fresh and contain antigen in sufficient concentration to provoke a response. Also, it is advisable that test solutions of adequately prepared and purified allergic substances, rather than groups of substances, should be used so that reasonable specificity of the tests is ensured.

The common antigens used routinely in the tests include inhalants: grass, tree, shrub and flower pollen; moulds such as cladosporium, neospora, penicillium, *Apergillus fumigatus*, etc; house dust and house dust mite; animal hair and dander; birds' feathers such as canary and budgerigar; various vegetable fibres such as cotton and kapok. Also various foods such as cow's milk casein and lactalbumen; egg yolk and egg white; nuts and fruits; meats and fish. To this routine list can be added solutions and extracts made from any antigen that may be indicated during history taking.

Method. There must be no preliminary cleansing of the skin.

The volar aspect of the forearm is most frequently the site of the tests, but in very young children, the skin of the back can be used.

A small drop of solution is placed on the skin, and the skin pricked by needle through the drop. There should be no bleeding, which, indeed, would invalidate the test. The method is similar to that of smallpox vaccination. An identifying mark is made.

After a few minutes, usually 5 to 15, a positive reaction is shown by an area of erythema surrounding the prick site, with a weal in the centre. The size of the weal appears to be related to the degree of hypersensitivity.[16] The weal-and-flare reaction usually disappears after half to two hours. However, in some cases, notably housedust mite sensitivity and sensitivity to budgerigars and other birds as well as some moulds, a late reaction may occur some 2 to 24 or 48 hours later. While the weal-and-flare reaction is Type I (immediate hypersensitivity), the late reaction is probably Type III (Arthus hypersensitivity). For this reason it is advisable to ask the child to keep the identifying marks undisturbed for at least 24 hours after the tests have been carried out. The size of the reactions should be measured in millimetres only. Recording of reactions as +, ++ or +++ is subjective and inaccurate and thus of little value.

Nasal and Bronchial Provocation Tests

Many workers believe that testing the effect of antigens at the target sites relates more reliably than skin tests to the symptoms (rhinitis, asthma).[10,15,17] However, doubts do exist of their greater value,[18] and there are doubts concerning the ethics of inducing possibly severe asthma and/or rhinitis in a child who must be hospitalised for the test. Furthermore, positive reactions need not necessarily show that the particular antigen is responsible for the child's usual symptoms. In addition, non-specific reactions may occasionally occur.

With the above reservations, the tests are usually carried out as follows[10]: the solutions are as those used for skin testing, although it seems advisable to omit the phenol preservative which can irritate the bronchial mucosa.[15] No antihistamines or any other drugs should be administered for 24 hours before the test and the test should only be carried out during a period of full remission. Prior to the provocation tests, pulmonary function tests should be performed (FEV_1, FVC and PEFR as routine).

For *bronchial provocation* a nebuliser is used, starting with small doses of the antigen and increasing the concentration but not so much as to produce non-specific irritation of the respiratory epithelium.[10] Positive results are shown by evidence of bronchial constriction, cough, hypersecretion, and marked reduction (20 per cent or more) of FEV_1, FVC and PEFR; often, also rhinitis, and often after a few hours also, pulmonary and nasal secretions which are rich in eosinophils.[10] It is necessary to be prepared to treat any severe asthmatic attack or anaphylaxis that may arise from the tests.

No more than one antigen should be tested at any one time and on any one day. Preferably there should be an interval of at least one day between tests.

Nasal provocation is performed by using one nostril for the test and the other nostril as control. One drop of the test solution is placed in the nose, positive reactions arising within a few minutes. These consist of sneezing, mucosal reddening and swelling, with hypersecretion. Here also, one test on any one day should be the rule, and the nostrils should be used alternately. Occasionally, an attack of asthma is provoked.

As with skin testing, reactions may be of immediate Type I; but there may also be later Type III reactions with the same range of antigens (q.v.). This biphasic response could be a partial explanation of those cases of asthma that respond at first to adrenaline, but which, after relief, relapse and fail to react to further doses of adrenaline.[19] A concise account of the bronchial provocation tests regarding methods, technique and scope has been written by Aas.[23]

Specific Precipitating Antibodies

Specific precipitating antibodies may be found in the serum of some patients who suffer from 'bird-fancier's' lung (sensitivity to birds such as pigeons, budgerigars and parrots), and in the serum of those sensitive to *Aspergillus fumigatus*, and possibly other moulds. Some of these patients show Type I reactions in the skin, but many do not, so that careful search may be necessary.[19] These antibodies are evidence supporting the diagnosis of Type III hypersensitivity, probably mediated by IgG antibodies.

In recent years an *in vitro* test for detecting anti-IgE circulating antibodies has come into increasing use. This is the RAST (radio-allergosorbent test),[20] which is based on the following facts—

1. Allergens of different types can be chemically coupled to Sephadex.
2. These polymer-coupled allergens retain their capacity to bind antibodies of the IgE class.

3. Even when bound these antibodies can further bind anti-IgE antibodies.
4. The anti-IgE antibodies can be purified and labelled with radioactive isotopes.

The test is allergen specific and is also IgE-specific.

RAST correlates highly with the results of bronchial provocation tests (90 to 96 per cent) and moderately well (60 to 85 per cent) with skin tests.[20,24–27] Results are recorded as + or ++ if radioactivity uptake is two to five times normal or greater, respectively. Serum can be stored at 20°C until analysed, and results can be obtained within 24 hours.

With the foregoing systematic approach, it should be possible to determine allergic factors in asthma in at least 80 per cent of children. However, there remains a small proportion in whom difficulty arises. These are nearly all the children whose illness is precipitated by, or occurs in close association with a non-specific respiratory tract infection. While about 50 per cent of asthmatic children relate their asthma to 'infection', most of them can be proved to have an allergic basis.

Many children are classified as *wheezy bronchitics* from a very early age, often as young as three months, simply because they wheeze when they develop a respiratory infection. The major difficulty has been to determine whether these attacks are really infections or whether they are manifestations of immunological reaction. There have been reports of an association between asthma and infection (*see* Chapter 2). Infection, especially when repeated, causes a loss of ciliated mucosal cells in the bronchi which contributes to the difficulty of eliminating the glairy mucus produced during an attack, thus increasing respiratory embarrassment.[21] The older infant and young child arriving for a first consultation have often been pre-labelled as suffering from 'wheezy bronchitis'. It would be well to realise that there may be a continuous spectrum of illness from the mild wheezy bronchitis at one end of the scale to asthma at the other.[22]

Differential diagnosis may also be difficult in the very young child, as this is the age at which many otherwise normal children develop various respiratory infections. It is also essential to exclude—

Cystic Fibrosis,
Hypogammaglobulinaemia,
Alpha—1 antitrypsin deficiency,
Bronchiectasia,
Chronic adenoidal infection,
Foreign body in bronchus,
Congenital heart disease,

External compression of trachea, e.g. enlarged lymph nodes, vascular anomalies.

The most important factor in diagnosis is physician-awareness. The association of the illness with eczema, a family history of allergic illness, evidence of hypersensitivity, eosinophilia of blood, nasal and bronchial secretions, the tendency to complete remission between attacks, and the recognition of trigger factors should all help to point in the direction of a diagnosis of asthma.

Complications of asthma in children

Status asthmaticus is the most important and serious complication of asthma because, if not adequately and promptly treated it can lead to the death of the child.

Pulmonary collapse-consolidation.
Ribcage deformity (pigeon-breast, barrel-chest, Harrison's sulcus).
Pulmonary eosinophilic infiltration (caused by infection with *Aspergillus fumigatus* most commonly).[19]
Bronchiectasis.
Pneumothorax.
Traumatic emphysema; rupture.
Cor pulmonale.
Compensatory polycythaemia.

The last four of these complications are rare, but it is important to recognise their possible occurrence.

References

1. Chai, H., Purcell, K., Brady, K. and Falliers, C. J. (1968) Therapeutic and investigational evaluation of asthmatic children. *Journal of Allergy*, **41,** 1, 23.
2. Knowles, G. K. (1973) Pulsus paradoxus as valuable sign of severity of asthma. *Lancet*, **2,** 1356–9.
3. Chasin, W. D. (1973) Current Paediatric Therapy (Ed. Gellis and Kagan), Vol 6, p. 106. Philadelphia: W. B. Saunders.
4. Taylor, B., Evans, J. N. G. and Hope, G. A. (1974) Upper Respiratory Tract in Cystic Fibrosis. *Archives of Disease in Children*, **49,** 133.
5. Delaney, J. C. (1973) Asthma, nasal polyposis and aspirin sensitivity. *Annals of Internal Medicine*, **79,** 761.
6. Kuzemko, J. A. (Personal Communication).
7. Simon, G., Connolly, N., Littlejohns, D. W. and McAllen, M. (1973) Radiological abnormalities in children with asthma and their relation to the clinical findings and some respiratory function tests. *Thorax*, **28,** 115.
8. Turk, J. L. (1969) *Immunology in Clinical Medicine*, p. 27 London: Heinemann.
9. Morrow Brown, H. (1973) Abstracts, Charles Blackley Centenary, Symposium, Nottingham.

10. Aas, K. (1969) Allergic asthma in childhood. *Archives of Disease in Childhood*, **55,** 1.
11. Gell, P. G. H. and Coombes, R. R. A. (Ed.) (1968) *Clinical Aspects of Immunology*, 2nd ed. Oxford: Blackwell.
12. Ishizaka, K., Ishizaka, T. and Holbrook, M. M. (1966) Correlation of reaginic activity with gama-E globulin antibody. *Journal of Immunology*, **97,** 840.
13. Parish, W. E. (1970) Short term anaphylactic IgG antibodies in human sera. *Lancet*, **2,** 591.
14. Bryant, D. H., Burns, M. W. and Lazarus, L (1973) New type of allergic asthma due to IgG 'Reaginic' antibody. *British Medical Journal*, **4,** 589.
15. Girard, J. P., Horvat, L. and Didsheim J. C. (1973) Inhalation tests as a routine diagnostic procedure in allergic asthma. *Annals of Allergy*, **31,** 597.
16. Stenius, B., Wide, L., Semour, W. M., Holford-Stevens, V. and Pepys, J. (1971) Clinical significance of specific IgE to common allergens. *Clinical Allergy*, **1,** 37.
17. Colldahl, H. (1967) Inhalation tests in allergy diagnoses. *Acta Allergologica*, 22 Suppl., **7,** 3. Copenhagen.
18. Falliers, C. J., (1972) Pulmonary and adrenal effects of alternate-day corticosteroid therapy. *Journal of Allergy and Immunology*, **49,** 6, 365.
19. Pepys, J. (1973) Abstracts, Charles Blackley Centenary Symposium, Nottingham.
20. Wide, L., Bennich, H., and Johannsson, S. G. O. (1967) Diagnosis of allergy in an in vitro test for allergen antibodies. *Lancet*, **2,** 1105.
21. Dunnill M. S. (1971) *Pathology of Asthma*. Ciba Foundation Study Group No. 38, p. 38. London and Edinburgh: Churchill Livingstone.
22. McNicol, K. N. and William, H. B. (1973) Spectrum of asthma in children. *British Medical Journal*, **4,** 7.
23. Aas, K. (1975) *The Bronchial Provocation Test*. Springfield, Illinois: Thomas.
24. Stenius, B. and Wide, L. (1969) Reaginic antibody (IgE) skin and provocation tests to Dermatophagoides culinae and house dust in respiratory allergy. Lancet, **2,** 455.
25. Apold, J., Havnen, J., Hvatum, M., Oseid, S. and Aas, K. (1974) The radioallergosorbent test (RAST) in the diagnosis of reaginic allergy. *Clinical Allergy*, **4,** 401.
26. Wide, L. (1973) Clinical significance of measurement of reaginic (IgE) antibody by RAST. *Clinical Allergy*, **3,** 583.
27. Bryant, D. H., Burns, M. W. and Lazarus, L (1975) The correlation between skin tests, bronchial provocation tests and the serum level of IgE specific for common allergens in patients with asthma. *Clinical Allergy*, **5,** 145.

CHAPTER 7

Emergency Treatment

Jan A. Kuzemko

IF IT IS to be comprehensible the treatment of an illness so protean in its manifestations and so obstinately persistent in its duration as asthma needs to be split up and considered in the forms in which the illness commonly presents. Hence, here it will be discussed under the headings: the acute attack that does not amount to status, status asthmaticus, and minor exacerbation.

The Acute Attack

This may be an acute attack of asthma in a child suffering from intermittent asthma or an acute incident in a case of continuous asthma.

It would perhaps not be out of place at this point to describe an acute attack. There is a sudden or perhaps a more gradual onset of wheezing, usually accompanied by breathlessness, and often preceded by a dry cough, which occurs very frequently during the night or early morning. Examination shows a marked over-use of the accessory muscles of respiration, severe hyperinflation, with difficulty in expelling air from the lungs, and considerable limitation of air excursion. There may be cyanosis of lips or face. Percussion will usually reveal generalised hyperresonance. Auscultation reveals poor air entry and excursion which may be localised, lobar or generalised. High-pitched rhonchi, especially in expiration are very widespread. However, bronchial obstruction may be severe and so limit air movement that there is insufficient excursion to produce rhonchi. This could lead to misjudgement of the severity of the attack.

Treatment of the acute asthmatic attack at home

Undoubtedly, the most effective drug is still adrenaline. A subcutaneous injection of a solution of adrenaline 1 in 1,000 should be given slowly. The dose should be 0·1 to 0·3 ml, depending on the age of the child. If the response is partial or nil, the dose can be repeated after a ten minute interval for three doses only. Great care should be taken that adrenaline is not given together with other bronchodilators as the cumulative effect may predispose to cardiac arrhythmia.

Terbutaline has been used as a subcutaneous injection and the results are satisfactory.[14] The dose is 0·01 mg/kg up to the maximal dose of 0·25 mg/kg. The duration of action is usually about four hours.

In some small children, instead of adrenaline the effect of aminophylline suppositories (5 mg/kg) can be tried. The child's progress should then be observed for the next 30 minutes. Orally administered aminophylline may be equally effective since blood levels following rectal or oral dosages are similar.[16]

Whatever measures are taken, it is most important to stay with the child until definite improvement occurs. It is cruel, and bad judgement to leave a breathless child partly treated, such neglect usually leading to status asthmaticus.

Oral corticosteroids for acute attacks at home. The use of oral corticosteroids outside hospital practice is regarded with some misgiving by many doctors, for these agents are very potent and can produce numerous undesirable effects if used indiscriminately. Nevertheless, they are life-saving and, in many children with an acute attack of asthma, can help to terminate an episode quickly and reduce suffering to a minimum. If the doctor cannot end an attack quickly with a parenteral bronchodilator, his choice is clear—either the child should be admitted to hospital or he should use oral corticosteroids early, in pharmacological doses, and review progress every few hours. It should be remembered that the normal physiological replacement dose of cortisone acetate in children is 0·7 mg/kg per 24 hours (the prednisolone dose is 1/5th the cortisone dose). A satisfactory pharmacological dose of prednisolone is 2 mg/kg per 24 hours.

The following scheme is recommended—

(*a*) Make sure there is no underlying infection; if one is suspected give the appropriate antibiotic.

(*b*) Make sure the family can cope at home and that they understand all your instructions.

(*c*) Write down all your instructions clearly.

(*d*) Administer hydrocortisone hemisuccinate (i.m. or i.v.) 100 mg, and start on oral prednisolone.

Example: Boy, weight 25 kg, No. of tablets—prednisolone 5 mg.

Day	a.m.	mid-day	p.m.
1	4	3	3
2	2	2	2
3	1	1	1
4	1	0	1
5	1	0	0

Such a scheme can be modified depending on circumstances, weight and age of the child, duration of illness, etc.

(*f*) If the child has been treated with sodium cromoglycate or steroid aerosol, discontinue these for two days. Many children will stop anyway because they experience difficulties in inhaling and bronchospasm will prevent any satisfactory particle dosage being deposited in the airways, most of the drug thus being swallowed and of no benefit whatsoever.

(*g*) The child's progress should be reviewed in six hours.

(*h*) The parents should be firmly instructed that if they become concerned about the child's condition at any time they should telephone the doctor immediately or, failing that, take the child to the Casualty Department of the nearest hospital. There should be no delay.

If the child does not respond fairly quickly to these simple measures then he should be admitted to hospital as he will almost certainly require oxygen therapy for hypoxaemia and, often, correction of acid-base disturbances and intravenous fluid therapy for dehydration.

Management of the acute attack in hospital

Investigations required immediately on admission

(*a*) Electrolytes, blood urea and haematological values.

(*b*) Blood PaO_2, $PaCo_2$, ph and gases.

(*c*) X-ray of chest. Portable X-ray is at times preferable. There should be a minimum of delay.

Action. Start oxygen therapy with high humidity at once. A mask is not often tolerated by a child, hence, a tent must be used. If so, the oxygen flow should be at least 8 to 10 litres per minute to reach an ambient oxygen concentration of about 35 per cent in as short a time as possible. Some of the oxygen devices and their performance are shown in Table 7.1. The aim is

Table 7.1 Performance of Oxygen devices

Type of device	Oxygen flow litres/min.	Concentration %	Comment
Tent (child)	8–10	60–80	Useful for upper airway humidity.
Tent (adult)	10–15	40–50	As above
Face Tent	4–8	30–45	Best for very young and humidity.
Face mask	4–8	35–65	Variable dead space.
Venturi Mask (24%)	4	24	Very useful
Nasal catheter or cannula	4	40–55	Not well tolerated.

to administer oxygen concentrations fairly accurately with a minimum effective dead space.

Intravenous fluid therapy. Depending on the child's clinical state, this should be started early rather than late. An intravenous drip provides an easy and painless means of administering drugs and antibiotics. If the child is dehydrated because of recurrent vomiting or fever, intravenous fluids should be given immediately, e.g. 1·8 g/litre saline or 43 g/litre dextrose are satisfactory solutions. Amounts should be calculated on a 24 hour basis and allowance made for any degree of dehydration.

Guidelines

Age in years	Solution ml/kg
0–1	150
1–2	120
2–3	100
4–6	90
7–12	70
Over 12	50

Aminophylline. The doctor should ascertain what drug treatment the child has had during the last six hours. If the patient has had adrenaline and oral bronchodilators, it is useful at this stage to give intravenous aminophylline as an infusion drip (5 mg/kg) over a 4-hour period. Pierson and colleagues[9] administering aminophylline 7 mg/kg by rapid intravenous infusion, followed by a slow infusion of 9 mg/kg for 24 hours demonstrated a significant improvement in ventilation in a group of 23 children. Others recommend administering the total calculated 8-hour dose within 15 minutes.

Intravenous salbutamol. It has been shown that in adults[21,22] slow (2 to 5 minutes) intravenous injection of 250 μg salbutamol, repeated if necessary 15 minutes later may be very effective in the treatment of an acute attack. Our experience of this method in children is very limited.

Antibiotics. In the presence of infection or suspected infection, a broad spectrum antibiotic should be given. It can be given either orally, if the child is not too ill, or intravenously. Frequent intramuscular injections in the young child are not only painful but upsetting. We have found a combination of ampicillin and cloxacillin very effective. If the child is sensitive to one of the penicillins, erythromycin should then be used.

The majority of children will improve with this simple standard treatment. As breathing improves, help in eliminating sputum can be obtained by physiotherapy and postural drainage. Subsequent treatment can be administered orally.

Inhalation therapy. We have little experience in using isoprenaline or salbutamol aerosols in the treatment of acute attacks, a form of treatment that is popular in some centres in Canada and the United States[1]. Dilutions of the appropriate bronchodilator (in normal saline) are given over a short period of time. However, it should be remembered that, on occasions, aerosols will not only be ineffective but will result in accentuation of hypoxaemia.[12,13]

Status Asthmaticus

A child is considered to be in status asthmaticus if his acute attack of asthma has failed to show sustained improvement within two hours of admission to hospital. A retraction of the sternocleidomastoid muscle strongly suggests severe airway obstruction.[8] Ineffective treatment may lead to death or hypoxic brain damage.[15]

Corticosteroids. There are two facts every doctor should remember when using corticosteroids for the management of status asthmaticus. Firstly, he should use large doses at the onset in order to raise the level of plasma cortisol to 150 to 200 micrograms per 100 ml at least. It has been shown that clinical improvement rarely occurs if the levels are below that figure.[1,2] Secondly, the beneficial effects of such treatment will only be apparent in 4 to 6 hours. It is for this reason that the attending doctor should, immediately following the child's admission, decide whether or not he needs to use corticosteroids. When in doubt it is safer to use them rather than wait. Prednisolone given orally will show maximum effect at 9 to 12 hours, some beneficial effect at 3 hours, and none after 36 hours; whereas some beneficial effects from intravenous hydrocortisone can be observed at 1 hour and at a maximum of 5 hours. The following is the scheme we use—

	Hydrocortisone hemisuccinate
Children under 2 years of age	200 mg initially 100 mg every 3 hours
2–5 years	250 mg initially 100 mg every 2 hours
5–12 years	300 mg initially 150 mg every 2 hours
Over 12 years	400 mg initially 200 mg every 2 hours.

Collins and his colleagues,[19] studying adults, suggested a dosage of 3 mg/kg body weight of hydrocortisone every six hours as a continuous intravenous infusion after an initial loading dosage of 4 mg/g intravenously.

Pierson and colleagues[1] showed that early treatment of status asthmaticus with corticosteroids (betamethasone, hydrocortisone or dexamethasone) caused significant improvement in arterial hypoxaemia which was independent of any changes in pulmonary function.

Since corticosteroids may cause hypokalaemia, it is important to use supplements of potassium chloride at the rate of 20 mmol/litre to each 400 ml of i.v. fluid and obtain periodic E.C.G. readings (1 gram KCl = 13 mmol of K and 13 mmol of chloride).

The mode of action of corticosteroids in status asthmaticus remains undetermined.[2] Most likely they exert their effects by anti-inflammatory properties, by increasing intracellular cyclic AMP, by preventing the formation of histamine in mast cells—which appears to be one of the major substances released during asthmaticus[3–6]—and by restoring sensitivity of the bronchial muscle to catecholamines (endogenous or exogenous), thus facilitating bronchodilatation.[20]

Other measures

The results of the initial investigations on admission should be now available, therefore—

(a) Correct acidosis if present. The bicarbonate dose (mEq/litre), as recommended by Astrup and colleagues[7] (base deficit $\times$ 0·3 $\times$ body weight in kg = mmol required for complete correction). 1 gram of sodium bicarbonate contains 12 mmol of bicarbonate and 12 mmol of sodium (84 g/litre or 1 mmol/ml).

(b) Decide if the child is hypoxaemic. His clinical state may suggest this. He may be restless and confused and have tachycardia. If on admission his PaO_2 was low (below 85 mmHg or 11·3 kPa) and $PaCo_2$ above normal (35 to 45 mmHg or 4·65 to 6·0 kPa), check the value again. A rising $PaCo_2$ implies imminent respiratory failure. It is vital to rely on clinical judgement rather than on blood gases alone as these may or may not be accurate.

(c) Examine chest X-ray. Exclude pneumothorax.

Respiratory failure

We follow the criteria laid by Downes[11] and colleagues with some modifications—

(*a*) Severe inspiratory gasps are taken.
(*b*) Breath sounds are almost inaudible.
(*c*) Chest movements poor.
(*d*) Consciousness is disturbed.
(*e*) Cyanosis, despite 40 per cent oxygen administered for 10 minutes.

If any of the two criteria are present, the child should immediately be transferred to the Intensive Care Unit, for almost certainly assisted ventilation will be needed and the services of a skilled anaesthetist required.[17]

In our experience, only the occasional child in status asthmaticus requires assisted ventilation and hardly any bronchial lavage.

Sedation

In general, sedatives have little place in the management of the child in an acute attack or status asthmaticus. It must be remembered that all sedatives cause respiratory depression, which may further aggravate hypoxaemia. In the occasional, emotionally disturbed child a quick and short acting sedative such as chloral hydrate is best. Distress of hypoxaemia must not be confused with emotional disturbance—wrong judgement and wrong treatment will soon become apparent.

Physiotherapy

It is important to discuss with the physiotherapist the child's clinical state, treatment and measures to be undertaken. Once there is definite improvement very gentle postural drainage should be started in order to facilitate the opening of smaller airways and removal of secretions. No attempts should be made to alter the child's rate of breathing since the respiratory centre not only adjusts his depth of breathing but also its rate so that he can obtain the most effective ventilation using as little effort as possible.[23]

Management of Minor exacerbation

Slight exacerbations of asthma not amounting to any distress will usually respond to rest and the administration of a bronchodilator. Salbutamol either as a syrup, tablet or aerosol is most effective. Relief usually occurs in 10 to 20 minutes. Most episodes will subside with the above treatment. If a minor degree of airway obstruction is still present in two to three hours, it is useful to continue bronchodilators for the next 24 hours. Six-hourly dosages should be used. Failure to respond to such measures usually implies a concurrent upper or lower respiratory tract infection.

One of the reasons why children fail to respond to these simple and conventional treatments is that parents are not given clear instructions. We have found it advantageous to write the instructions down for them and to ask them to follow the same scheme every time the child has a minor episode. With such a scheme, the majority of parents can deal effectively with minor episodes themselves. Successful management of minor episodes will build up confidence towards coping with more serious situations should they arise and thus learning in depth about their child's asthma.

References

1. Pierson, W. E., Bierman, C. W. and Kelly, V. C. (1974) A double-blind trial of corticosteroid therapy in status asthmaticus. *Pediatrics*, **54,** 3, 282.
2. Avideo, D. M. and Carrillo, L. R. (1970) Antiasthmatic action of corticosteroids: A review of the literature on their mechanism of action. *Journal of Clinical Pharmacology*, **10,** 3.
3. Schayer, R. W., Smiley, R. L. and Davis, K. J. (1954) Inhibition by cortisone on the binding of new histamine in rat tissues. *Proceedings of the Society for Experimental Biology and Medicine*, **87,** 590.
4. Logson, P. J., Middleton, E. and Coffey, R. G. (1972) Stimulation of leucocyte adenyl cyclase by hydrocortisone and isoproterenol in asthmatic and non-asthmatic subjects. *Journal of Allergy and Clincial Immunology*, **50,** 45.
5. Cline, M. J. and Melmon, K. L. (1966) Plasma kinins and cortisol: A possible explanation of the anti-inflammatory action of cortisol. *Science*, **153,** 1135.
6. Eberlein, W. R., Bongiovanni, A. M. and Rodriguez, C. S. (1967) The complications of steroid treatment. *Pediatrics*, **40,** 279, 1967.
7. Astrup, P., Jorgensen, K., Siggard-Anderson, O. S. and Engel, K. (1960) The acid-base metabolism: A new approach. *Lancet*, **1,** 1035.
8. McFadden, E. R., Kiser, R. and DeGroot, W. J. (1973) Acute bronchial asthma: Relationship between clinical and physiological manifestations. *New England Journal of Medicine*, **288,** 221.
9. Pierson, W. E., Bierman, C. W., Stamm, S. J., and Var Arsdel, P. P. (1971) Double-blind trial of aminophylline in status asthmaticus. *Pediatrics*, **48,** 642.
10. Masselli, R., Casal, G. L., and Ellis, E. F. (1970) Pharmacologic effects of intravenously administered aminophylline in asthmatic children. *Journal of Pediatrics*, **76,** 777.
11. Downes, J. J., Wood, D. W., Stiker, T. W. and Lecks, H. I. (1966) Diagnosis and treatment: Advances in the management of status asthmaticus in children. *Pediatrics*, **38,** 286.
12. Palmer, K. N. V. and Diament, M. L. (1967) Effect of aerosol isoprenaline on blood gas tensions in severe bronchial asthma. *Lancet*, **2,** 1232.
13. Van Metre, T. E. (1969) Adverse effects of the inhalation of excessive amounts of nebulised isoproterenol in status asthmaticus. *Journal of Allergy*, **43,** 101.
14. Sly, M. R., Badiei, B., Faciane, J. (1975) Treatment of acute asthma in children with subcutaneous terbutaline. *Journal of Allergy and Clinical Immunology*, **55,** 97.
15. Bierman, C., Pierson, W., Shapiro, G. and Simons, E. (1975) Brain damage from asthma in children. *Journal of Allergy and Clinical Immunology*, **55,** 2, 126.
16. Lillehei, J. P. (1968) Aminophylline—oral v· rectal administration. *Journal of the American Medical Association*, **206,** 530.
17. Downes, J. J., Fulgencio, T. and Raphaely, R. (1972) Acute Respiratory Failure in infants and children. *Pediatric Clinics of N. America*, **19,** 2, 423.
18. Ellul–Micallef, R. and Fenech, F. F. (1975) Intravenous prednisolone in chronic bronchial asthma. *Thorax*, **30,** 312.
19. Collins, J. V., Clark, T. J. H., Brown, D. and Downsend, J. (1975) The use of corticosteroids in the treatment of acute asthma. *Quarterly Journal of Medicine*, **44,** 259.
20. Shenfield, G. M., Hodson, M., Clarke, S. and Paterson, J. W. (1975) Interaction of corticosteroids and catecholamines in the treatment of asthma. *Thorax*, **30,** 430.
21. Spiro, S. G., Johnson, A. J., May, C. S. and Paterson, J. W. (1975) Effect of intravenous injection of salbutamol in asthma. *British Journal of Clinical Pharmacology*, **2,** 495.
22. May, C. S., Paterson, J. W., Spiro, S. G. and Johnson, A. J. (1975) Intravenous infusion of salbutamol in the treatment of asthma. *British Journal of Clinical Pharmocology*, **2,** 503.
23. Gandevia, B. (1959) Pulmonary function and physiotherapy. *Australian Journal of Physiotherapy*, **5,** 87.

CHAPTER 8

Long-term Management

Jan A. Kuzemko and S. Bedford

CARING FOR THE asthmatic child in remission is a long-term procedure requiring frequent and close supervision. Fortunately, several treatments available enable most children to lead normal or near normal lives. During remission full assessment of the child should be made.

About two hours is spent initially with each new child and his family. Asthma and its management are freely discussed. A plan of action is agreed upon and written instructions regarding any treatment given. Each child is then reviewed in two to four weeks and then periodically, but not less than four times a year.

Response to treatment. A daily record card of symptoms and twice daily records of the peak expiratory flow rates (PEFR) give valuable information and should be routine. It is of great value to ask the parents (or the child) to keep a record for two to three weeks before any active treatment is given. The observations will serve as a base-line, and any response to therapy such as bronchodilators, sodium cromoglycate, or steriod aerosols can then be judged subjectively (symptoms) and objectively (PEFR). Figure 8.1 illustrates a typical example.

Treatment

(a) Bronchodilators. If the attacks are infrequent, mild in nature, and do not interfere with the child's activities, all that is required is periodic administration of a bronchodilator such as salbutamol or terbutaline (for dosage *see* Appendix and review on pages 79 to 88).

Many children are prescribed bronchodilators unnecessarily, for far too long and, often, prophylactically between infrequent attacks. At times two or even three bronchodilators are used simultaneously. Such polypharmacy is to be condemned. It is our experience that written instructions are essential if the parents are to understand clearly what is required of them. Knowledge of one established bronchodilator, its actions and side-effects will serve the doctor far better than a superficial grasp and use of many

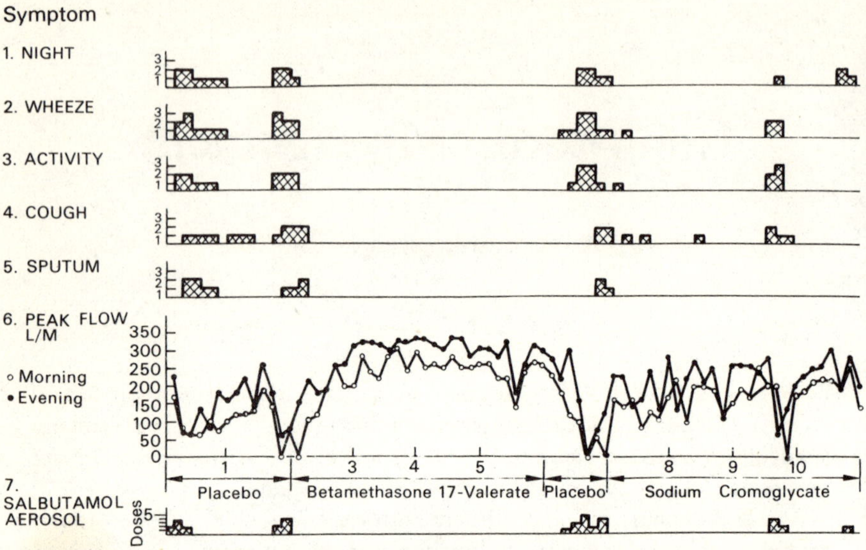

Fig. 8.1 A summary of subjective and objective observations in an 11-year-old boy with asthma during a 12-week period, which strongly suggests that the patient fared best on a betamethasone 17-valerate aerosol

fashionable agents of doubtful additional therapeutic value.

(b) Sodium Cromoglycate. Frequent episodes associated with atopy and allergy can best be prevented by using sodium cromoglycate, a full review of which is given on pages 88 to 98. This drug is most helpful in children subject to frequent episodes because it not only reduces the number and severity of attacks, but also relieves the dyspnoea and cough associated with exercise. It is a prophylactic agent and should be administered continually over a long period of time once it has been found effective in the individual child. Apart from occasional dryness of the throat and cough after inhalation, it appears to be free from side-effects. Each capsule contains 20 mg of sodium cromoglycate in lactose base. Following inhalation, about 10 per cent of the drug is retained in the spinhaler, 30 to 50 per cent is deposited in the mouth, about 10 per cent enters bronchi and lungs, and the rest is swallowed and appears unchanged in faeces. Only about 4 per cent of the drug is actually absorbed from the lungs.[29,30]

The majority of children over the age of three years can inhale sodium cromoglycate effectively, and many under the age of three do equally well. It is a fallacy that children under four to five years of age cannot take sodium cromoglycate satisfactorily. We have looked at this problem in our group of asthmatic children under the age of four, a summary of our conclusions being set out in Tables 8.1, 8.2 and 8.3. Age and sex distributions are shown in

Table 8.1 Distribution of age and sex

Age Range	Number of boys	girls	Total
2·0 years to 2·6 years	3	1	4
2·7 years to 3·0 years	6	6	12
3·1 years to 3·6 years	10	5	15
3·7 years to 4·0 years	19	4	23
Total	38	16	54

Table 8.2 Distribution of period of treatment with sodium cromoglycate

Time on sodium cromoglycate	No. of children
6 months to 1 year	23
1 year to 2 years	14
2 years to 3 years	6
Over 3 years	11
Total	54

Table 8.3 Results before and after sodium cromoglycate

	*Number of instances during			
	the year before drug started†	1st year of drug therapy†	2nd year of drug therapy**	3rd year of drug therapy††
Home visits by G.P.	110 (2·0)	6 (0·1)	4 (0·1)	2 (0·1)
Hospital Admissions	28 (0·5)	2 (0·0)	3 (0·1)	1 (0·1)
Corticosteroid periods	28 (0·5)	0	0	0
Bronchodilator periods	31 (0·6)	0	0	0

* Averages per patient in brackets:
† Based on sample of 54 for year before and first year after.
** Based on sample of 31 for second year after.
†† Based on sample of 17 for third year after.

Table 8.1, Table 8.2 shows the distribution of period of treatment with sodium cromoglycate, and Table 8.3 the results of treatments before and after administration of sodium cromoglycate. The results were assessed using the following criteria—

1. Exacerbation requiring a home visit from a general practitioner.
2. Emergency admission to hospital.
3. Continuous use of oral corticosteroids over a period of four weeks or longer.
4. Continuous use of bronchodilators for a period of four weeks or longer.

There can be little doubt that this group of young children derived great benefit from the drug.

It takes time and patience to teach the very young child how to inhale sodium cromoglycate effectively. On occasions we supply the young child with an empty spinhaler or even with a DeBono whistle. The spinhaler is introduced and talked of as a toy, e.g. a whistle. A long time is spent in instructing the parents and the child in its use. At times, two spinhalers are supplied to the family, one for the mother and father to 'play with' and the other for the child. Once the child accepts an empty spinhaler it is relatively easy to persuade him to use it loaded. As a rule it takes up to a week to get the child to take the drug regularly. It is our experience that a child can empty a capsule with two to three inhalations. If he needs more attempts, either his technique is wrong or he has some degree of bronchospasm preventing him from taking the full breaths rapidly. In the latter case he can be helped by administering a bronchodilator, waiting for about 20 minutes, and then trying the spinhaler again.

The dosage of sodium cromoglycate usually recommended is one capsule four times a day, but it is our experience that if the child uses his spinhaler correctly, and if he obtains little or no benefit, then increasing the dose from twice daily will not produce a corresponding improvement. However, Konig and Godfrey[1] have found that in children who do not respond to two or four capsules, increasing the dose to six capsules daily may sometimes be of benefit.

It is essential for the doctor to maintain efficient supervision to be sure that the child is using the spinhaler correctly. The majority of asthmatic children show marked improvement, figures varying from 50 to 75 per cent in different centres.[2–4] In our clinic, the overall improvement is approximately 75 per cent over both short and long term periods of treatment.[5]

Children who have been treated for various periods of time with oral corticosteroids or ACTH can often be successfully weaned from these after treatment with sodium cromoglycate is firmly established. At times, some will relapse. Such children may have to return to oral corticosteroids, but many can, and should be transferred to steriod aerosols. There may remain a few who require both oral corticosteroids and steroid aerosols for the successful control of their asthma, but the rationale for using both on long-term basis is founded on the whim of the doctor rather than any sound evidence. Failure to respond to sodium cromoglycate calls for a re-appraisal of the management and assessment of the child.

After a child has been relatively symptom free for at least one year, we try to discontinue sodium cromoglycate. Experience of the first 20 children who satisfied such criteria and stopped their treatment is worth discussing here: 12 have remained symptom free during the subsequent four years (last assessment) but 8 relapsed within one month, were poorly controlled on bronchodilators, and returned to sodium cromoglycate treatment. They have remained well since then.

It is disputed whether sodium cromoglycate has a persistent 'carry over' effect. We support the contention of Silverman and his colleagues[6] that 'carry over' effect does not exist. Most of our children have relapsed within the first few days.[7] Thus, in attempting to wean a child from sodium cromoglycate it is advisable to reduce the dose gradually, perhaps taking three to four weeks to complete the change.

In the infant who is unable to take sodium cromoglycate effectively, dilutions of the drug in a solution (20 mg in 2 ml of aqueous s.) have been used with some success. A special power-operated nebuliser (e.g. Wright's) at a flow rate of 6 to 8 litres a minute through a face mask is required. In some young children, incorporating a whistle (which whistles only when the child inhales) to the spinhaler is effective in persuading the child to use it.

And what about the future? It is hoped that chemists will be able to alter the structure of sodium cromoglycate to make it effective by mouth, which would widen its scope and acceptability.

(c) Steroid aerosols. If the child is not gaining benefit from sodium cromoglycate, it is rational to try the effects of steroid aerosols such as betamethasome dipropionate or betamethasone-17-valerate before any oral corticosteroids are considered. The majority of children over the age of three years can inhale the aerosol successfully. Both are dispensed in canisters containing approximately 200 doses, and are administered by the pressurised metered aerosol delivering 50 and 100 μg per puff respectively. The dose in children is two puffs (100 and 200 μg respectively) two to four times a day. Children who become well controlled can be managed very effectively with four puffs, given either in the morning or evening. This simplifies therapy considerably and ensures that the drug is taken.[44] If a child is not responding to conventional doses of oral corticosteroids, he is unlikely to respond to steroid aerosols, and vice versa. We know of no study that has disproved this observation. A comprehensive review of the steroid aerosols is given on pages 98 to 110.

As with all forms of aerosols therapy, it is essential that the technique of administration is learned thoroughly, and is a further reason for adequate and frequent supervision.

(d) Corticosteroids and corticotrophin. There remain some children with asthma who derive insufficient relief from sodium cromoglycate and the other methods of treatment described, and are unable to lead normal or near normal lives, which must be the aim of any management. These

children may benefit from an oral corticosteroid such as prednisolone. The usual regime is to start with relatively high doses, e.g. 5 mg four times a day, to maintain this level until there is improvement, and then gradually reduce the dose in small steps until the lowest dose that will suppress attacks is reached. The aim is to maintain treatment at this low level and, if possible, to stop the corticosteroids completely within a short period of time. By this method some children will need their corticosteroids only in the event of a severe attack that will not respond to other methods of treatment. Administration would thus be intermittent. However, there are still some children who require continuous corticosteroid therapy and in this group there always exists a real danger of causing suppression of the hypothalamo-pituitary-adrenal system (HPA), with its attendant interruption of growth, cushingoid facies, fluid retention, weight gain, possible hypertension and poor response to stress such as operation or accident, infection, diabetic state, etc. These ominous complications are strictly dose related and can be minimised by keeping the dose of prednisolone below 5 mg/day.[8] Equivalent doses of other corticosteroids in common use are shown in Table 8.4. As there is a 'carry over' effect with corticosteroids, it is reasonable to try alternate day treatment,[9,10] which minimises the suppression of the HPA system.

Table 8.4

	Equivalent dose (mg)
Hydrocortisone	20
Prednisolone	5
Prednisone	5
Methyl-prednisolone	4
Triamcinolone	4
Betamethasone	0·75
Dexamethasone	0·75

During long-term treatment with corticosteroids it is essential that the state of the HPA system should be frequently assessed, which is achieved most simply by the tetracosactrin screening test. Tetracosactrin is a synthetic corticotrophin that, when injected intravenously or intramuscularly, rapidly increases the amount of circulating cortisol if the HPA system is intact. The method and its interpretation have been fully described elsewhere.[8,9] In any child on continuous corticosteroid drugs, it is imperative to carry out tetracosactrin tests every three or four months.

ACTH is an alternative to oral corticosteroids. It is administered intramuscularly, and doses vary between 10 and 80 units. A short and long acting ACTH is available. As with corticosteroids, there is a 'carry over' effect with ACTH and its substitutes, hence the drugs can be given at intervals of 48 hours without minimising their beneficial effect in many, but not all, children.

Some investigators have shown that ACTH and the synthetic corticotrophins suppress growth less than do corticosteroids[11,12,34] and it should be remembered that asthma itself can be responsible for growth retardation.[35] Nevertheless, therapeutic doses for long periods of time have no advantage over corticosteroids as far as growth is concerned,[13,14,31] as is shown in Figs 8.2 and 8.3.

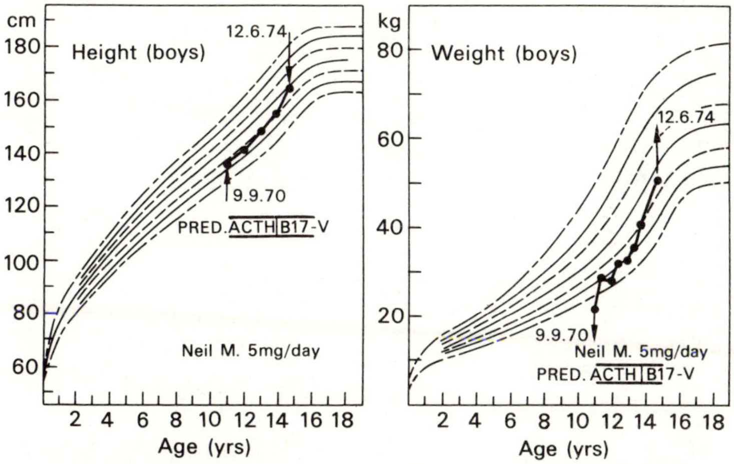

Fig. 8.2. Height and weight pattern of an asthmatic boy on 5 mg prednisolone daily, then ACTH 20 units twice weekly and subsequently betamethasone-17-valerate aerosol

When withdrawing corticosteroids after long-term use, it is vital that they be reduced very gradually, taking several weeks or even months to achieve complete withdrawal. The adrenal glands are suppressed during therapy and they may take a long time to recover, even if there is a change over to ACTH. Adrenal function must be assessed with great care before reducing the dose of corticosteroids to below maintenance level. This warning is necessary owing to the fact that it is now possible to replace corticosteroids with either sodium cromoglycate or steroid aerosols.

Finally, children on oral corticosteroids should carry a *steroid warning card* at all times.

Hyposensitisation

Throughout the world a vast literature on the subject of hyposensitisation has been published since Noon's paper on 'Prophylactic inoculation against hay fever' appeared.[15] In a critical review of this measure, Wittig[16] lays down

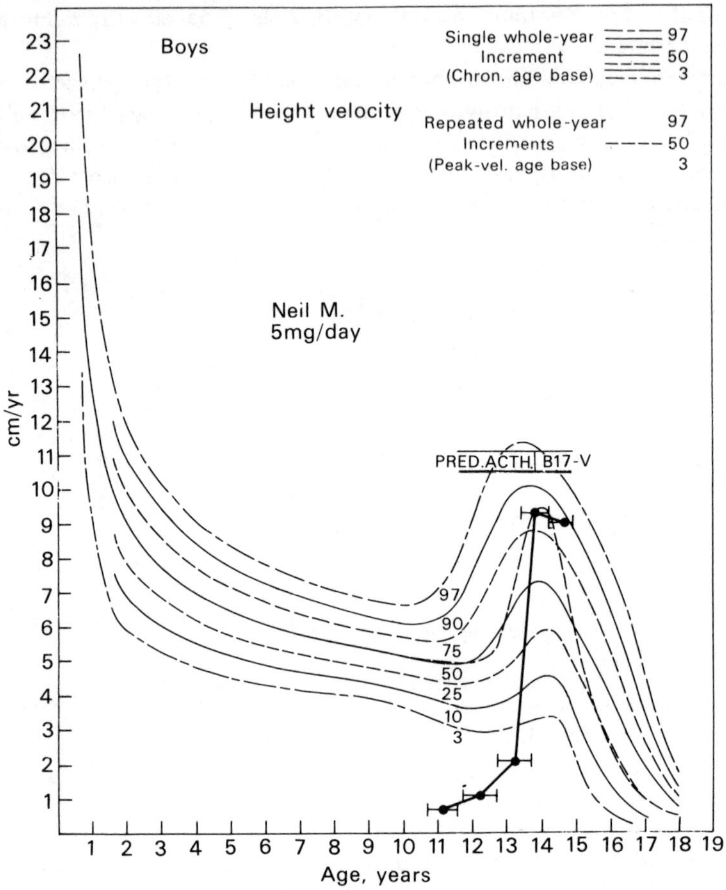

Fig. 8.3 Growth velocity of an asthmatic child showing minimal growth on 5 mg prednisolone daily or ACTH gel 20 units twice weekly and growth spurt on change of therapy to betamethasone-17-valerate aerosol. (Some growth spurt may have been due to puberty but throughout observation genital growth has remained at Stage I. Tanner's classification)

the criteria to be fulfilled before undertaking this method of treatment. These are—

(*a*) The presence of an allergic disorder.
(*b*) A demonstrable allergen.
(*c*) Absent alternative pathogenetic mechanisms.
(*d*) Identification of contributory psychological factors.
(*e*) A monitoring system regarding the safety and effectiveness in each patient who is to receive prolonged injection therapy.

In adults this lists should be considered comprehensive, but in children with asthma additional difficulties arise. The age of the child, and the most recent advances in drug treatment must be considered, and weighed against the trauma of subjecting the child to injections over a period of years with the constant possibility of anaphylactic reactions to his injections from which he may or may not gain prolonged benefit.

A long-term prospective study of the value of prolonged hyposensitisation therapy in children, with a follow up of 14 years, was carried out by Johnstone and Dutton.[17] They reported considerable success, especially in the group of children with perennial asthma receiving the highest concentrations of allergen. Twenty-two per cent of the control group and 71 per cent of the treated group had 'lost' their asthma by their 16th birthday.

There is conflict of opinion regarding the age at which it is reasonable to start hyposensitisation. Some workers (mainly American) treat at a very early age, even as young as two years of age. Others will not use the method in children under the age of ten, believing that many children will improve spontaneously anyway, and that the need for frequent and painful injections is of doubtful value.

The best results occur in those children suffering from seasonal asthma (pollen determined) or seasonal hay fever. In planning treatment it is important to time the course of therapy so that the last injection is given shortly before the allergen season begins. With this scheme about 25 per cent of the children will benefit as regards their asthma, but up to about 80 per cent in cases of hay fever.

The offending allergen is given weekly by subcutaneous injection, starting with a small dose and increasing with each weekly injection until a peak dose is reached at which reactions occur. The injection that follows is of the same strength as the one prior to the reaction, a dose level that is continued weekly for 4 to 8 weeks. The next four injections are given at two-weekly intervals and are then followed by monthly doses at the same concentration. This schedule is continued monthly (or perhaps, later on, even six-weekly) for a long time, perhaps several years, the period depending on the outcome of sensitivity tests (skin, provocation, RAST, etc). When it is demonstrated that the patient's reaction to challenge with the offending allergen is either absent or greatly reduced, injections are stopped.

Reactions produced in the patient by the injections are local (at the injection site) or general (anaphylactic) and may be mild or severe. At the point of injection there may be erythema, itching, swelling or wealing (Type I reaction). The anaphylactic reaction can be severe enough to threaten life. Treatment of the reaction, if severe enough to warrant it, should be with Soln. Adrenaline 1/1000, given subcutaneously and slowly in a dose of 0·2 to 0·5 ml. Response is usually rapid. Because of these reactions, it is advisable to keep the child under observation for at least half an hour after he has been given his injection. It is possible to inhibit most of these reactions by prior administration of oral antihistamine drug.

The solutions of allergens for hyposensitisation are aqueous, pyridine-extracted alum-precipitated, or oil suspended. The best results occur with aqueous solutions, but the untoward reactions are more frequent and more severe than with the alum-precipitated solutions. The oil suspensions are almost obsolete now because of the problem of irregular absorption. A method of hyposensitisation by means of intranasal allergen solutions has been used and appears to be of some benefit in allergic rhinitis, although of doubtful value in asthma.[18]

The house dust mite and asthma. Many workers in the field of allergy and asthma are convinced that the house dust mite (*Dermatophagoides farinae* or *D. pteronyssinus*) plays a large part in causing asthma attacks, especially in children.[19–21] The house dust mite lives in a warm, damp environment and its main food appears to be shed skin scales. These accumulate maximally in bedding and may account for some children having asthma attacks in the early hours of the morning. It has been observed that one mite (i.e. about 1 μg of allergen) can provoke bronchospasm.[39] Protection for these children (and all children who show positive sensitivity reactions to the mite) can be much aided by vacuum cleaning the bedclothes, floor and window coverings of the bedroom and periodic exposure of the bedding to bright sunlight which destroys both the mite and its antigenicity. The following are simple, written instructions we give to parents—

Measures to reduce the population of the house dust mite in your home

1. All rooms
   (*a*) Vacuum clean thoroughly at least once a week (including armchairs, settees, etc)
   (*b*) Keep your furniture as free from dust as possible.
2. Child's bedroom
   (*a*) Vacuum clean room twice weekly.
   (*b*) Use all bedding made of synthetic material only.
   (*c*) Change sheets and pillow cases weekly.
   (*d*) Use light easily washable curtains.
3. Air bedding in direct sunlight as often as weather permits.
4. If you keep household pets, e.g. dog, cat, use a special shampoo periodically.

Sarsfield and colleagues[40] have confirmed in a detailed study of 14 children with mite-sensitive asthma that such avoidance measures were very effective in reducing significantly the incidence of attacks. Such procedures, therefore, should be adopted in the first instance with any mite-sensitive child before resorting to hyposensitisation. A non-toxic fungicidal and bactericidal spray is being tried but it is too early to assess results.[41]

Much work has been done with various extracts of mite in skin sensitivity and nasal and bronchial provocation testing, RAST, etc. In our experience about 80 per cent of asthmatic children will show positive hypersensitivity reactions to the house dust mite in the skin and with RAST. Although it is possible by hyposensitisation procedures to lower or even abolish this hypersensitivity, it does not necessarily lead to an improvement in the child's asthma. Hyposensitisation to the mite allergens has been shown to be of limited success in a short-term trial[36] although much better results can be obtained if the injections are continued for a long time,[37] perhaps years, as the relapse rate is very high.[38]

The media used for presenting the house dust mite allergens are, aqueous solutions, pyridine-extracted, alum-precipitated, oily suspensions and tyrosine absorbed.

Psychological status

It has been stressed during history-taking that the psychological background of asthmatic children is important. During the long-term follow up of children with asthma, many changes both of soma and psyche may occur, especially in relation to the results of treatment. The child who is relieved of his acute attacks of incapacity with their attendant limitations of activities is a much more relaxed child in all ways. His mother takes part in this improvement as do all the other members of the family. In general, the home becomes a much happier place.

However, some children do not improve enough for them to lead normal lives, partly because medication is only partially effective and partly because of the family situation and because the general psychological state of the child and his family have not improved. There are parents who are over-protective or ambivalent or rejected, or there may be poor interparental relationships. There may be single parent homes, or parents may have separated and the child is 'pulled' both ways. In these circumstances, it is imperative that attempts be made to ascertain the background of the situation and, with the help of various social services, assistance in straightening out the difficulties should be offered. In such cases, it is of value to enlist the help of a child psychiatrist whose expertise may illuminate the obscurity and uncertainties of the situation. His assessment of the child and the parents could be of help in the otherwise refractory case. In general, the occasions when psychiatric assistance is required are strictly limited.[33]

Asthma Clinics

Our experience leads us to conclude that asthmatic children are best treated in out-patient clinics specially provided for the purpose. That children offer problems differing considerably from those of adults must be recognised which inevitably leads to the suggestion that adults' and childrens' clinics should be separated. Attacks of asthma in children may arise with little warning and reach alarming proportions very rapidly. In order to help both patient and parents, the services of physician and staff should be freely available day and night. Psychologically, therefore, the clinic should be part of a general hospital physically, administratively and with regard to staff.

If the child develops an acute attack or even if the mother thinks one is developing, it is essential that hospital admission should be available freely and with minimal delay. What matters most is the continuity of management and treatment by a permanent team rather than by frequently changing doctors with little experience of, or interest in, asthma. Any ethical difficulties that may arise when bypassing the family doctor in this way can nearly always be ironed out by prior discussion between the hospital doctor and the family physician.

To establish the closest rapport with the child patient and his parent, it is necessary to have frequent consultations and to provide adequate time for the fullest discussions of any associated problems. During such consultations all aspects of the child's illness should be freely talked about, in this way building up a relationship which usually guarantees that any treatment prescribed will be carried out fully. It must be remembered, too, that supervision may have to be continued for several years, a fact reinforcing the necessity of establishing mutual confidence.

Hypnotherapy

Hypnosis as a method of treatment of asthma has been used for many years. After all, suggestion plays a part in many forms of medical treatment and its efficacy, therefore, can be exploited for the relief of symptoms. Many studies have claimed a symptomatic relief. Objective controlled studies are few. Morrison-Smith and Burns[22] in a group of 25 children studied for a period of one month, failed to show that hypnosis was beneficial, and in another study[23] it was shown that with daily autohypnosis, little improvement occurred in the first month of treatment. However, a controlled study of 252 patients,[24] of whom one-third were under the age of 19 years, showed beneficial value of hypnotic methods. Also, physicians who had previous experience in the use of hypnosis achieved better results than those without any previous training.

Undoubtedly there is a place for hypnosis and psychotherapy in selected children with asthma. The best results are obtained in children lacking confidence in themselves, those who are over-anxious and insecure, and those who have been indiscriminately and half-heartedly subjected to various forms of treatment and, as a result, have, with their parents, abandoned faith in their therapeutic value. Hypnosis should be considered an adjunct to other forms of treatment.

It is our view that a doctor who treats children with asthma and who has no working experience of hypnosis is missing an opportunity of being able to help some of his patients. It is beyond the scope of this book to describe in detail patient selection, methods of induction, and the phenomena of hypnosis; for details, the reader is referred elsewhere.[25]

Before starting treatment, full discussion with both parents and the child should be held. Common misapprehensions and beliefs regarding hypnosis should be explained. It is not recommended to practice hypnosis with children younger than six years of age because lack of attention may cause problems in achieving satisfactory induction. It is essential to teach the child autohypnosis for the treatment to be most successful and this should be started as early as possible during a course of therapy.

If patient selection is good, results of treatment can be very gratifying and well worth the time and effort, as is illustrated by the two examples below—.

Case I

A.B., a girl of 10 years 9 months was first seen when the family moved to the area. She had long-standing asthma dating from the third year of life. Despite numerous drugs, including long-term oral corticosteroids and/or ACTH, she continued to have symptoms every few days. In fact, since starting school she had never completed a full week and had to be admitted to various hospitals on numerous occasions because her asthma could not be controlled at home. Family history, negative. Her parents were very concerned about the child's illness but well adjusted and co-operative. They welcomed and sought help from many doctors of various medical disciplines but improvement in their child's asthma had always remained very short lived. Attempts at boarding school education failed because the child 'spent most of her time in the sick-bay rather than the class room'. When seen she was grossly cushingoid and stunted in linear growth. Withdrawal of all drugs resulted, surprisingly, in an asthma-free interval of three months duration but was followed by frequent exacerbations, as in the past. Re-appraisal of her treatment and frequent supervision were only partly successful. In view of the failure of drugs to control her symptoms and despite negative psychiatric history, it was felt that hypnotherapy might be of value. Her response to this has been satisfactory. She has remained relatively well during two years of observation but for the infrequent minor exacerbations that were easily relieved by a short course of bronchodilators. Her growth pattern and weight loss has been equally impressive. Her school attendance has been excellent.

Case 2

C.D., a boy aged 8 years 3 months, has had asthma since the age of four years. On average, his parents had consulted their doctors at least 20 times a year since that time. Although he had many episodes of asthma, each one had always been characterised by a sudden onset of severe bronchospasm and, equally, each could be satisfactorily managed by injection of adrenaline, aminophylline, or a very short course of oral corticosteroids. Preventive measures (drugs and environment) to control his asthma were judged to have failed. The boy obtained most relief from bronchodilator aerosols which he excessively over-used despite attempts by many doctors to limit their use. Although one has had suspicion of some interfamily problems these were denied by the parents and none were uncovered by psychiatrists. A school report was partly helpful and pointed out that 'the boy rarely joins in games because of his asthma and spends most of his time being a linesman'. The decision to use hypnotherapy was taken jointly with the parents and the boy, following his admission to hospital in a severe status asthmaticus. The results of treatment throughout 18 months of observation has remained satisfying to all. Apart from oral bronchodilators, which the boy takes before prolonged exercises, he leads a normal life.

We believe that there is a place for hypnotherapy in selected children with asthma and that the best doctor to use this form of treatment should be a physician who is actively engaged in treating children with asthma and who is fully aware of its benefits and limitations.

Ancillary Services and School Activities

As the asthmatic child is often called upon to perform physical exercises at school, it is important to enlist the aid and co-operation of his teachers. The child may need to be excluded from all exertion in the early stages of treatment while, later on, he may need the administration of pre-exercise drugs to help him carry out normal activities. There should, therefore, be good communication between physician, parent, child and teacher.

Various social services are available in most countries to help individuals in their relationship within the community. These could be of considerable benefit and help especially in dealing with poor housing conditions, in helping parents of poor intelligence to carry out the prescribed treatment, and in coping with broken home situations where there is only one parent.

In these cases, the good community worker can be a most valuable link between the patient and the clinic services.

Residential schools: 'parentectomy'. The removal of the asthmatic child from the home and his parents (so-called parentectomy) is said by some to be a useful therapeutic measure. It is undoubtedly true that a short-term admission to hospital gives both the child and his parents a break from one another and can sometimes be of value.

The decision to admit a child with asthma to a special residential school is often an arbitrary one and not dictated by the child's clinical condition. In a review of admissions of pupils with various handicaps to residential establishments, Pless, Rackham and Kellock[42] found that 50 per cent of the asthmatic children were sent away because their parents had financial, social or emotional problems, although there did not appear to be any acute deterioration in the child's asthma. Medical and educational factors were significant in 20 per cent and 25 per cent of the children respectively. Moreover, requests for admissions varied from county to county—those areas with organised medical, social services and educational departments rarely made use of residential schools.

The problems of educating children with various degrees of ability in small residential schools have been recently reviewed.[43] The facilities for primary school education were on the whole adequate, but the secondary school children were often required to attend local schools in the area because not all subjects were satisfactorily taught at the residential school.

Little is known regarding the optimum time an asthmatic child should spend at a residential school to obtain the best all-round benefit, or how many children eventually readjust and are able to attend ordinary schools near their homes. Of 9 asthmatic individuals known to us who attended residential establishments between the ages of nine and twelve only 3 were able to return to ordinary schools after two years. There was little improvement in their asthma. The other 6 continued at residential schools until 16 years of age. Of these 6, 1 died at the age of 22 years during an attack of asthma, 3 require medical supervision, and the remaining 2 are symptom free.

Residential schooling should be considered where there are serious emotional problems in the family as a result of which the child's educational attainments become seriously impaired. It is of little value to send a child away for less than two years, and this aspect should be fully discussed with the parents. The choice of school should be based on its academic excellence rather than on its 'homely' atmosphere. Adequate medical facilities should be fully available day and night. The decision should be taken jointly and in consultation with the educational authorities, social services, the family doctor and the paediatrician. The parents and the child should be invited to visit a selected school which should be known to at least one responsible member of the team. The parents should be given ample opportunity of airing their impressions of the school and declining the offer if they should be unhappy about any aspects.

The authorities concerned in making the decision to send a child away from home have a duty to meet periodically with the parents and the child in order to discuss his general and educational progress. As Pinkerton and Weaver[26] pointed out, such separations of the child from his parents should be designed to repair relationships rather than to destroy them. Dispatching a child for a vague period of time to an unknown school far away from his home and family so that local services 'can get a rest' is to be condemned. Such a decision in the long run creates more problems than it solves.

Lastly, it has never been established whether the long-term stay at a residential school is of any lasting benefit to the individual and his family; on the contrary it has been suggested that the death rate of young asthmatic people who have lived in residential schools is higher than that of the general population.

An American experience of long-term hospital care of asthmatic children has been reviewed recently by Sadler.[32] The conclusions are very indefinite.

Breathing Exercises

The value of breathing exercises during an attack of asthma is undetermined. If they help the patient to relax and he is convinced of their benefit, they should be encouraged but never insisted upon.

Livingstone and Gillespie[27] first observed that breathing exercises between attacks were of possible value in the asthmatic individual. Numerous reports have since appeared suggesting that such exercises were of subjective benefit. Also, it has been suggested that a conditioning programme to improve the child's physical fitness is of value. Most of the exercises performed are based on those described by the Asthma Research Council and are of two types—

(*a*) Breathing exercises aiming at using specific muscles of respiration.
(*b*) Physical fitness exercises.

Breathing exercises aim to improve ventilation, to correct postural deformities, e.g. kyphosis, round shoulders, and to improve chest expansion. Most of the breathing methods aim at abdominally assisted respiration in which a conscious voluntary effort to increase intra-abdominal pressure by contracting the abdominal muscles is encouraged, thus increasing the expiratory force and moving the diaphragm as high as possible into the chest. Undoubtedly, exercises producing muscle relaxation, increased flexibility of the shoulder girdle and increased mobility of the thorax will result in improved posture. Some children may derive psychological benefit from such exercises and others who can perform breathing exercises skilfully can help themselves in a bout of bronchospasm. This may relieve anxiety and give the child increased confidence. It must be remembered, however, that many children with asthma dislike breathing exercises as they make them breathless—hence they should not be imposed on them without proper discussion and assessment. Description of the various breathing exercises is beyond the scope of this book for which the reader is referred to the Asthma Research Council Monogram.[28]

Physical fitness exercises

An asthmatic child whose disease is poorly controlled often leads a lonely and solitary life. Many of these children would like to participate in games, especially at school, but the fear of post-exercise bronchoconstriction is such that they sacrifice outdoor activities for the sake of apparent well-being. Moreover, many parents insist on abandonment of any games at school, since they have seen their child exhausted and breathless on numerous occasions when he has arrived home.

A scheme of physical activity in the asthmatic child can achieve a higher level of physical fitness than the child is able to attain beforehand. Such exercises do not alter the underlying pathological processes but they do increase muscular and cardiovascular efficiency so that the amount of work they do can be done at a smaller oxygen cost—thus reducing cardiac output and increasing cardiac reserve. Moreover, psychological benefits may also occur. Graded short exercises of two or three minutes duration are best. Exercises that promote the learning of new skills and the acquiring of greater muscle strength are useful. In this respect field events are strongly to be recommended. Short bouts of swimming are equally helpful in many children, because they improve co-ordination in breathing, encourage physical development and prevent chest deformities. Interestingly enough, singing lessons are equally helpful.

Prolonged uninterrupted exercises of 15 or more minutes are poorly tolerated by the asthmatic child. It is important to discuss this aspect with the mother, the child, and the teacher. In these situations, post-exercise bronchoconstriction can be almost completely prevented by the prior administration of a bronchodilator such as salbutamol which should be taken 20 minutes before an exercise or games. Steroid aerosols and corticosteroids have no effects on post-exercise bronchoconstriction.

Asthma, operations and corticosteroids

As a rule, children with asthma have no problems with anaesthesia. It is vital to ascertain the child's drug therapy. If he received prolonged corticosteroids which were stopped less than three months before a proposed operation, or is currently being treated with corticosteroids we use the following scheme—

(*a*) For simple procedure, e.g. tooth extraction, a single dose of 2 mg/kg cortisone injection B.P. is given intramuscularly.

(*b*) For a minor operation, 2 mg/kg cortisone injection B.P. is given 6 hourly for 24 hours by intramuscular injections.

(*c*) For a major operation, 2 mg/kg cortisone injection is given 6 hourly for 72 hours and then followed up with an oral dose of a corticosteroid, if required.

(*d*) For all critical emergencies hydrocortisone hemisuccinate, 2 mg/kg, is given intravenously as a single injection and then cortisone injections are followed as above.

Tests of the hypothalamic/pituitary/adrenocortical axis (H.P.A.) are not required. It takes about two months for the H.P.A. function to recover adequately following corticosteroid treatment.[45] The best single test of its function is the hypoglycaemia test.[46] Adrenocorticotrophin (ACTH) should not be used at the end of or during corticosteroid treatment since it impairs further the H.P.A. function although it reverses adrenal atrophy.[47]

Asthma and Immunisations

A child with asthma should not receive any active immunisation if he is recovering from an attack, other stressful illness, e.g. diarrhoea, or is on corticosteroids, immunoppressive agents or suffering from any illness affecting immunity.

Smallpox vaccination is contra-indicated in those children who have eczema, septic skin or recurrent rashes or who live with other children who suffer from similar disorders. Measles immunisation is well tolerated by the asthmatic child; if he is egg sensitive, a dog kidney or chick cell cultured vaccine should be used. With rubella vaccine there is even more choice—chick, duck, dog or rabbit. The value of combined measles–mumps–rubella vaccine remains undetermined. Poliomyelitis vaccine (Sabin type) is very safe. Immunisation against influenza should be confined to children with severe asthma.

There are no contra-indications to whooping cough vaccine and there is no point in using it after the age of five years. Diphtheria and tetanus vaccines are well tolerated and booster doses should be given every five years after primary immunisation. Immunisation against tuberculosis is free from any hazard and the policy laid down for U.K. school children should be followed, i.e. offered at about 13 to 14 years of age to tuberculin-negative individuals.

Passive immunisation against measles, using immunoglobulin from adult serum, should be considered in the ill child with chronic lung disease. It should be administered as early after exposure to the disease as possible, in the following doses—

Under 3 years–500 mg
Over 3 years—750 mg

Smaller doses than the above will attenuate an attack of measles and are unlikely to prevent it. Immunity lasts for three weeks or so. There is little to be gained by passive immunisation against other diseases, and in some cases, e.g. diphtheria and tetanus, there is always the risk of serum sickness or anaphylaxis.

Conclusion

Little is known of the extent to which a child with recurrent attacks of asthma causes disruption of daily family life. Undoubtedly, many families experience a great deal of difficulty in adapting to stresses such as disturbed nights, meals, school routine, work, etc. It is not surprising that such situations can cause tensions within the parents themselves and precipitate attacks of asthma in the child or even exacerbate new conflicts in the household. We have little doubt that proper control of asthma can diminish anxiety states to a significant degree.

An additional distress to parents is caused at times by a lack of readily accessible medical facilities. In the Isle of Wight study[48] about a quarter of parents experienced problems in obtaining immediate help. To what extent such failures lead to new anxieties in the parents and in the child is unknown, but is probably not insignificant.

We feel that the services outlined in this chapter may help in the management of the child with asthma and his family.

A high level of success in treating asthmatic children can be achieved only by dedicated application over a long period of time. The close relationship between the physician and his charge and the ability of the physician to utilise the services of anyone capable of helping, and to lead the team, are the basic units on which success is built. Increase in knowledge is preparing the way to increase relief for children suffering from this severe and often incapacitating illness, and is is therefore, the duty of the physician to keep himself abreast with the times and to be aware of recent advances in knowledge.

References

1. König, P and Godfrey, S. (1973) Effect of frequently administered DSCG in asthmatic children who previously responded poorly. *Clinical Allergy*, **3,** 395.
2. Smith, J. M. and Devey, G. F. (1968) Clinical trial of DSCG in treatment of asthma in children. *British Medical Journal*, **2,** 340.
3. Silverman, M., Connolly, N. M., Balfour-Lym, L. and Godfrey, S. (1972) Long term trial of DSCG and isoprenaline in children with asthma. *British Medical Journal*, **3,** 378.
4. Dickson, W. (1970) One year trial of Intal Co. on 24 children with severe asthma. In *DSCG in Allergic Airway Disease*. (Ed. Pepys J. and Frankland A. W.) London: Butterworths, pp. 105–119.
5. Bedford, S. and Kuzemko, J. A. (1970) Treatment of asthmatic children for 6 months with DSCG. *Clinical Pediatrics*, **9,** 12, 719.
6. Silverman, M. and Andrea, T. (1972) Time course of effect of disodium cromoglycate on exercise-induced asthma. *Archives of Diseases in Childhood*, **47,** 419.
7. Kuzemko, J. A., Bedford, S., Wilson, L. and Walker S. R. (1974) Sodium cromoglycate in children with reversible airways obstruction. *Postgraduate Medical Journal. Suppl.* 4, 50, 53.
8. Kuzemko, J. A. and Lines, J. G. (1970) Adrenal cortical function in children on steroids. *Archives of Disease in Childhood*, **45,** 215.
9. Kuzemko, J. A. and Lines, J. G. (1971) Adrenal cortical function in asthmatic children on alternate day steroids. *Archives of Disease in Childhood*, **46,** 366.
10. Walsh, S. P. and Grant, I. W. B. (1966) Corticosteroids in treatment of chronic asthma. *British Medical Journal*, **2,** 796.
11. Friedman, M. and Strang, L. B. (1966) Effect of long term corticosteroids and corticotrophins on the growth of children. *Lancet*, **2,** 568.
12. Brandon, M. L. (1972) ACTH v corticosteroids in therapy. *American Journal of Allergy*, **30,** 262.
13. Norman, A. P. and Sanders, S. (1969) Effect of corticotrophins on skeletal maturation and linear growth in six patients with severe asthma. *Lancet*, **1,** 287.
14. Kuzemko, J. A. (unpublished observations)
15. Noon, L. (1911) Prophylactic inoculation for hay fever. *Lancet*, 1572.
16. Wittig, J. H. (1970) Hyposensitisation therapy in allergic disease. *American Journal of Diseases of Children*, **120,** 58.
17. Johnstone, D. E. and Dutton, A. (1968) Value of hyposensitisation for asthma in children—a 14 year study. *Pediatrics*, **42,** 793.
18. Taylor, G. and Shivalkar, P. R. (1972) Nasal desensitisation. *Clinical Allergy*, **2,** 125.
19. Voorhorst, R. (1970) Quantitative aspects of the problem of house dust atopy and house dust mites. *Acta Allergologica*, **25,** 237.
20. Smith, J. M., Disney, M. E., Williams, J. D. and Goels, Z. A. (1969) Clinical significance of skin reactions to mites in children with asthma. *British Medical Journal*, **2,** 723.
21. Pepys, J., Chan, M. and Hargreave, F. E. (1968) Mites and house dust allergy. *Lancet*, **1,** 1270.
22. Morrison-Smith, J. and Burns, C. C. (1960) The treatment of asthmatic children by hypnotic suggestion. *British Journal of Diseases of the Chest*, **54,** 78.
23. Maher-Loughnan G. P., McDonald N., Mason A. A. and Fry L. (1962) Controlled trial of hypnosis in the symptomatic treatment of asthma. *British Medical Journal*, **3,** 371.
24. Maher-Loughnan, G. P. and Kinsley, B. J. (1968) Hypnosis for asthma—a controlled trial. A report to the Research Committee of the British Tuberculosis Association. *British Medical Journal*, **2,** 71.
25. Hartland, J. (1973) Medical and Dental Hypnosis and its Clinical Applications. 2nd edn. London: Bailliere Tindall.
26. Pinkerton, P. and Weaver, C. M. (1970) *Childhood Asthma in Psychosomatic Medicine*, 2. (Ed. O.W. Hill) London: Butterworths, p. 99.
27. Livingstone, J. L. and Gillespie, M. (1935) Value of breathing exercises in asthma. *Lancet*, **2,** 705.

28. Asthma Research Council: Exercises for asthma and emphysema. 3rd Revision. London.
29. Walker, S. R., Evans, M. E., Richards, A. J. and Paterson, J. W. (1972) The fate of ($_{14}$C) disodium cromoglycate in man. *Journal of Pharmacy and Pharmacology*, **24**, 525.
30. Moss, G. F., Jones, K. M., Ritchie, J. T. and Cox, J. S. G. (1971) Plasma levels and urinary excretion of disodium cromoglycate after inhilation by human volunteers. *Toxicology and Applied Pharmacology*, **20**, 147.
31. Wright, W. C., Siegel, S. C., Lippe, B. M. and Wong, S. R. (1974) Effects of synthetic ACTH on corticosteroid induced growth suppression. *Journal of Allergy and Clinical Immunology*, **53**, 52.
32. Sadler, J. E. (1975) The long term hospitalization of asthmatic children. *Pediatric Clinics of N. America*, **22**, 173.
33. Mattsson, A. (1975) Psychologic Aspects of childhood asthma. *Pediatric Clinics of N. America*, **22**, 77.
34. Drever, J. C., Malone, D. N. S., Grant, I. W. B., Douglas, D. M. and Lutz, W. (1975) Corticotrophin after corticosteroids in children with asthma and growth retardation. *British Journal of Diseases of the Chest*, **69**, 188.
35. Falliers, C. J., Tan, L. S., Szentivanyi, J., Jorgensen, J. R. and Bukantz, S. C. (1963) Childhood asthma and steriod therapy as influences on growth. *Americal Journal of Diseases of Children*, **105**, 127.
36. Taylor, B., Sanders, S. S. and Norman, A. P. (1974) Hyposensitization in childhood asthma. *Clinical Allergy*, **4**, 35.
37. Aas, K. (1971) Hyposensitization in house dust allergy asthma. *Acta Paediatrica. Scandinavica*, **60**, 264.
38. Abstracts of the 9th European Congress of Allergology and Clinical Immunology (1974). London: Pitman Medical.
39. McAllen, M. K., Assem, E. S. K. and Maunsell, K. (1970) House dust mite asthma. Results of challenge tests on five criteria with *D. pteronyssinus*. *British Medical Journal*, **2**, 501.
40. Sarsfield, J. K., Gowland, G., Toy, R. and Norman, A. L. E. (1974) Mite sensitive asthma of childhood. Trial of avoidance measures. *Archives of Disease in Childhood*, **49**, 716.
41. Penaud, A., Nourritt, J., Autran, P., Timon-David, P., Jacquet-Francillon, M. and Charpin, J. (1975) Methods of destroying house dust pyroglyphid mites. *Clinical Allergy*, **5**, 109.
42. Department of Education and Science (1972) Schools for Delicate Children. In *Aspects of Special Education*, p.2. Education Survey, 17. London: H.M.S.O.
43. *Aspects of Special Education*. (1972) Education Survey 17, p. 2. London: H.M.S.O.
44. Marshall, N., Walker, S. R. and Kuzemko, J. A. (unpublished observation)
45. Plumpton, F. S., Besser, G. M. and Cole, P. V. (1969) Corticosteroid treatment and surgery. *Anaesthesia*, **24**, 3.
46. James, V. H. T. and Landon, J. (1969) *Recent advances in endocrinology*, p. 50. (Ed. V. H. T. James) Edinburgh: Livingstone.
47. Donald, R. A. and Espiner, E. A. J. (1974) Plasma gonadotrophin response to gonadotrophin releasing hormone in patients with primary hypogonadism. *Journal of Clinical Endocrinology and Metabolism*, **39**.
48. Yule, W. and Rutter, M. (1970) *Education, Health and Behaviour*. (Ed. Rutter, M., Tizard, J. and Whitmore, K.) London: Longman, pp. 297–308.

CHAPTER 9

Recent Advances in Drug Therapy

S. R. Walker

THE TREATMENT OF reversible airways obstruction with pharmacologically active agents began in 1903 (Table 9.1) with the introduction of adrenaline. More than twenty years then elapsed before the first oral bronchodilator (ephedrine) was used in 1925. By 1938, theophylline was being utilised for its adrenergic effect and this was followed closely in the 1940s by combinations of theophylline with other therapeutic agents.

Table 9.1 Advances in the treatment of Asthma

1903	Adrenaline
1925	Ephedrine
1938	Theophylline
1948	Cortisone and ACTH
1950	Hydrocortisone and synthetic steroids
1957	Isoprenaline
1967	Salbutamol and Sodium cromoglycate
1972	Beclomethasone dipropionate
1973	Betamethasone valerate

Steroids revolutionised the treatment of asthma when they were first introduced in the early 1950s, and, were it not for their side effects, systemic steroids would be the therapy of choice today. In 1957, the adrenergic agonist, isoprenaline, was given by inhalation for the relief of bronchospasm and this was followed by the development of selective beta stimulants.

During the past few years there have been three major advances in the treatment of asthma—

1. Beta adrenergic drugs such as salbutamol and terbutaline, which act on the airways more selectively than isoprenaline and have a prolonged therapeutic effect;

2. Sodium cromoglycate, which acts prophylactically by blocking the mediators of antigen-induced bronchoconstriction;
3. Inhaled corticosteroids such as beclomethasone dipropionate and betamethasone valerate which also act prophylactically, providing steroid treatment but without producing systemic side effects.

I Bronchodilators

Pharmacological receptors. In order to classify bronchodilator drugs it is important to define certain pharmacological receptors. Although the general receptor hypothesis has its roots in the works of Langley, Ehrlich and Clark in the early 1900s it was not until the classical paper of Ahlquist[1] in 1948 that the concept of 'alpha' and 'beta' adrenergic receptors was introduced to explain the action of a series of sympathomimetic amines on various smooth and cardiac muscles. On the basis of the responses obtained, Ahlquist showed two different orders of potency. For the 'alpha' receptor the order was adrenaline, noradrenaline and isoprenaline; for the 'beta' receptor the order was isoprenaline, adrenaline and noradrenaline. The main responses to 'alpha' and 'beta' receptor stimulation in man are shown in Table 9.2.

Table 9.2 Responses to adrenergic receptor stimulation

Alpha	*Beta*
Broncho-constriction	Bronchodilatation
Vasoconstriction	Vasodilatation
Histamine Release Enhanced	Histamine Release Inhibited
Metabolic Effects	Metabolic Effects
	Cardiac Stimulation
	Skeletal Muscle Tremor

An important concept in the classification of beta adrenergic receptors was introduced by Lands and colleagues[2] in 1967. These workers were endeavouring to produce a beta stimulant that was more active on bronchial than on cardiac muscle. They stated that beta receptors could be divided into two types: $beta_1$ receptors which mediate the cardiac ionotropic and chronotropic effects, relaxation of intestinal smooth muscle and lipolysis; and $beta_2$ receptors which mediate the effects on bronchial smooth muscle, uterus, arteries, skeletal muscles, glycogenolysis and glycolysis. The possibility of selective stimulation of $beta_2$ receptors to relax bronchial smooth muscle, without the adverse $beta_1$ effects of cardiac stimulation, opened up a new line of research into drugs that might benefit asthmatic patients.

Classification of bronchodilator drugs

The principal bronchodilators are the sympathomimetic amines, and the structures of those commonly in use in the treatment of asthma are given in Fig. 9.1. They can be classified into three groups: those having—

(*a*) alpha and beta receptor activity:
adrenaline
ephedrine

(*b*) beta receptor activity only:
isoprenaline

(*c*) selective beta$_2$ adrenoreceptor activity:
orciprenaline
isoetharine
salbutamol
salmefamol
terbutaline
rimiterol

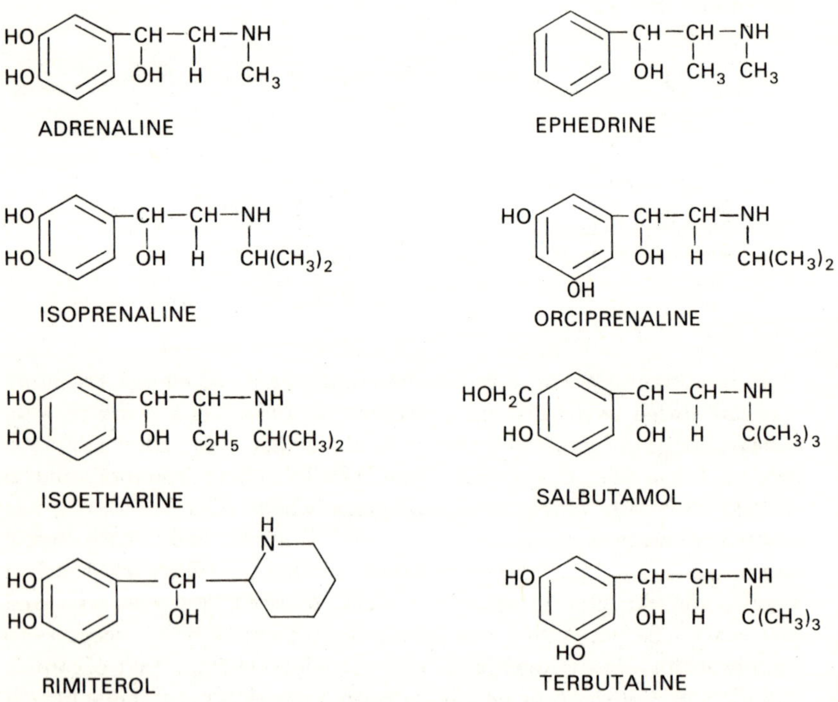

Fig. 9.1 Structures of some sympathomimetic amines

(*a*) *Stimulants of alpha and beta receptors. Adrenaline* is a naturally-occurring symphathomimetic amine. It has a short duration of action because its pharmacological effect is terminated by uptake into sympathetic nerve endings (uptake$_1$). It is inactive when given orally, being metabolised by both catechol-*o*-methyl-transferase and monoamine-oxidase in the gut and liver. Thus, adrenaline is effective only when given parenterally or by inhalation. Its use is usually confined to the treatment of status asthmaticus or severe attacks of bronchospasm. In addition to providing bronchodilatation, adrenaline also causes cardiac stimulation and vasoconstriction. Its alpha effect of vasoconstriction has been said to reduce mucosal oedema and thus contribute to its bronchodilator properties.

Ephedrine is structurally different from adrenaline (Fig. 9.1) in that it has lost the catechol grouping and is therefore resistant to catechol-*o*-methyl-transferase. Substitution of the methyl group at the alpha carbon atom means that ephedrine is also resistant to monoamine-oxidase. These two changes probably account for its longer duration of action and also for the fact that it is active orally. Because of its effect on central nervous stimulation it is often given in combination with a barbiturate. Methyl xanthines are sometimes included in this combination to reduce the bronchodilator dose of ephedrine required and, hence, the side effects. Ephedrine is thought to act by two different mechanisms: directly, in that it stimulates adrenoreceptors, and indirectly in that it releases catecholamines at sympathetic nerve endings. This indirect effect, which could lead to the depletion of noradrenaline, may explain why tolerance to the bronchodilator effect of this drug has been reported following continuous administration. Adrenaline and ephedrine both cause stimulation of the heart, resulting in tachycardia which increases the chance of arrhythmias.

(*b*) *Beta receptor stimulants. Isoprenaline* by inhalation was the most popular bronchodilator aerosol until the late 1960s. As can be seen (Fig. 9.1), it is structurally similar to adrenaline but the addition of an isopropyl group on the amine head results in a more potent beta effect on adrenergic receptors and an absence of alpha effects in man. This drug, following inhalation, gives rapid bronchodilatation but has a short duration of action (2 hours): it is rapidly removed from its site of action, being taken up into cells (uptake$_2$ mechanism for catecholamines). When isoprenaline is administered orally the majority of the dose is inactivated by being metabolised to an ethereal sulphate in the gut wall and, thus, is of little therapeutic use by this route.

As the pharmacokinetics of isoprenaline following inhalation and oral administration are similar, the implication is that the majority of an inhaled dose is swallowed. Dollery[3] has suggested that only about 10 per cent of a dose taken from a pressurised inhaler actually reaches the lungs, but this is sufficient to cause bronchodilatation. Paterson and colleagues[4] have shown that, when isoprenaline is given intravenously at various dose levels bronchodilatation and increase in heart-rate occur simultaneously; and so pharmacologically it is a non-selective beta receptor stimulant. However, it is made therapeutically selective by being administered directly to the lungs from a pressurised inhaler.

The dose of isoprenaline per puff from a pressurised inhaler varies from 100 μg to 500 μg in different preparations. Significant bronchodilatation has been observed in asthmatic patients[5] after a dose of 200 μg although no rise in pulse rate was recorded. However, it has been demonstrated that, using the 500 μg per puff preparation, the heart-rate rose in normal subjects when one to three puffs were administered.[6]

When considering the therapeutic benefits of the bronchodilators discussed so far the fact becomes clear the even isoprenaline has several disadvantages—

1. Its effect is short-lived;
2. It is inactive when given orally;
3. It activates $beta_1$ (cardiac) as well as $beta_2$ (bronchial) receptors.

The last disadvantage means that therapeutic doses of isoprenaline may be accompanied by cardiovascular effects such as tachycardia and arrhythmias. In addition, the ionotropic and chronotropic cardiac effects of isoprenaline cause an increase in the oxygen requirement of the heart, which is particularly undesirable in patients with heart disease or with more generalised hypoxia.

(*c*) *Selective $beta_2$ receptor stimulants. Isoetharine.* Lands and colleagues[2] carried out a systematic variation of the 'N substituent' of catecholamines in an effort to find a beta adrenergic receptor stimulant that would be selectively active on bronchial smooth muscle. This resulted in the discovery of isoetharine, which is about ten times as active on bronchial muscle as on cardiac muscle. This work also led to their hypothesis, which has already been mentioned, about the nature of beta receptors. Isoetharine is effective when given by inhalation and is available as an oral preparation. Although resistant to monoamine-oxidase it is metabolised in a similar manner to isoprenaline and, therefore, will have a short duration of action.

Orciprenaline. Repeated efforts to improve upon isoprenaline so as to produce a bronchodilator that would be selective and also longer acting has resulted in replacing the catechol function (which is responsible for the short duration of action of isoprenaline and isoetharine) by a resorcinol group, as in orciprenaline and terbutaline (Fig. 9.1). A resorcinol derivative is not inactivated by catechol-*o*-methyl-transferase, nor are these compounds likely to be actively transported through cell membranes. Orciprenaline, has a more prolonged duration of action than isoprenaline after inhalation and is also active orally. It is about 10 to 40 times less potent than isoprenaline in its pharmacological beta effects and is also essentially non-selective in its action.[7] Thus, the oral bronchodilator dose may cause a noticeable increase in heart rate.

Salbutamol. The best-known selective $beta_2$ stimulant is salbutamol. This bronchodilator is not susceptible to catechol-*o*-methyl-transferase or monoamine-oxidase, which may account for its prolonged duration of action. The hydroxymethyl group on the benzene ring prevents its conversion to an ethereal sulphate by sulphatases in the gut or liver and this compound is active by inhalation when given orally or intravenously. The N-tertiary butyl substituent in the side chain is associated with an increased $beta_2$ activity.[8] Following any route of administration, salbutamol is well absorbed, the majority of the dose being subsequently excreted in the urine.[9] Half that recovered from the urine is present as free salbutamol and the remainder as an unidentified metabolite.

Salmefamol. This drug is closely related to salbutamol. Animal experiments showed that it had better bronchodilator effect than salbutamol.[82] In man, effective bronchodilation can be observed up to four hours.[82] Whether it has similar effects on the blood pressure and heart rate as salbutamol remains undetermined.

Clinical studies have shown that salbutamol is as effective as isoprenaline in its bronchodilator activity while its duration of action is twice as long. Given by inhalation, salbutamol produces bronchodilatation for more than four hours; the response after oral administration lasts up to five hours. Following inhalation there are no systemic side effects, but after oral administration, skeletal muscle tremor is experienced by some individuals. The muscle tremor is a $beta_2$ effect; and separating bronchodilatation from the tremor-inducing activity of beta stimulants has not yet proved possible. Therefore, even the selective $beta_2$ stimulants should preferably be given by inhalation when appropriate. When given by inhalation in doses sufficient to cause bronchodilatation, salbutamol is hardly detectable in the blood; by contrast, significant blood levels of the drug must be reached with oral dosing before useful bronchodilatation is achieved.[9]

Terbutaline, a selective $beta_2$ stimulant, is a derivative of resorcinol with the same side chain as salbutamol (Fig. 9.1). It is poorly absorbed (25 per cent of the total dose) following either oral administration or inhalation.[10] It is metabolised to a sulphate conjugate but this occurs to a lesser extent than with the structurally-related isoprenaline, which may explain why the partially-absorbed terbutaline is a more effective oral bronchodilator than isoprenaline, even though the latter is completely absorbed when given orally. Clinical studies have shown that terbutaline produces adequate bronchodilatation following both inhalation and oral administration in doses that are without a significant effect on the heart rate. However, as with salbutamol, some patients experience tremor after oral doses of 5 mg or more.

Rimiterol is a member of a new series of sympathomimetic amines cyclised about the alpha carbon atom (Fig. 9.1). It is available only in aerosol form and has been shown to be as effective a bronchodilator as isoprenaline.[5] It is a specific $beta_2$ stimulant with a longer duration of action than isoprenaline but is shorter acting than salbutamol. It is metabolised in a similar manner to isoprenaline and is therefore inactive orally.[11]

Pharmacokinetics

Pharmacokinetic studies in man[9–11] with isoetharine, terbutaline, salbutamol and rimiterol have all confirmed that the metabolic pattern seen following inhalation is similar to that observed after oral administration. This indicates that the majority of an inhaled dose of these compounds is swallowed. However, the small proportion of the dose reaching the lungs acts locally to produce bronchodilatation without the adverse effects that may be seen when larger doses are given orally.

Mechanism of Action

The mode of action of beta adrenergic stimulants is shown in Fig. 9.2. Adenyl cyclase, the enzyme that catalyses the conversion of adenosine triphosphate (ATP) to cyclic 3′ 5′ adenosine monophosphate (cyclic AMP), is stimulated by beta adrenergic agonists. The cyclic AMP so formed mediates the cellular responses, resulting in bronchodilatation, vasodilatation, and inhibition of histamine release. Cyclic AMP is inactivated by hydrolysis to AMP, this reaction being catalysed by phosphodiesterases.

Methyl xanthines (theophyllines) also have an adrenergic effect by virtue of their inhibition of the phosphodiesterase enzymes which degrade intracellular cyclic AMP, thus potentiating beta adrenergic receptor stimulants. The theophyllines have also been shown to inhibit histamine release. Theophylline by mouth is variably absorbed and causes severe gastric irritation. However, choline theophyllinate and aminophylline are better absorbed and less irritant. In common with other beta stimulants, the methyl-xanthines can cause cardiac stimulation, vasodilatation and central nervous stimulation. They are often prescribed in combination with a sedative (barbiturates) in a compound tablet that also contains ephedrine. The theophyllines are thought to potentiate the effect of ephedrine, whereas the small amount of barbiturate is included to reduce the central nervous stimulation effect. The widespread acceptance of this polypharmacy probably stems from the apparent advantage that this combination offers of two bronchodilators in doses that are generally insufficient to cause the undesirable side-effects of either.

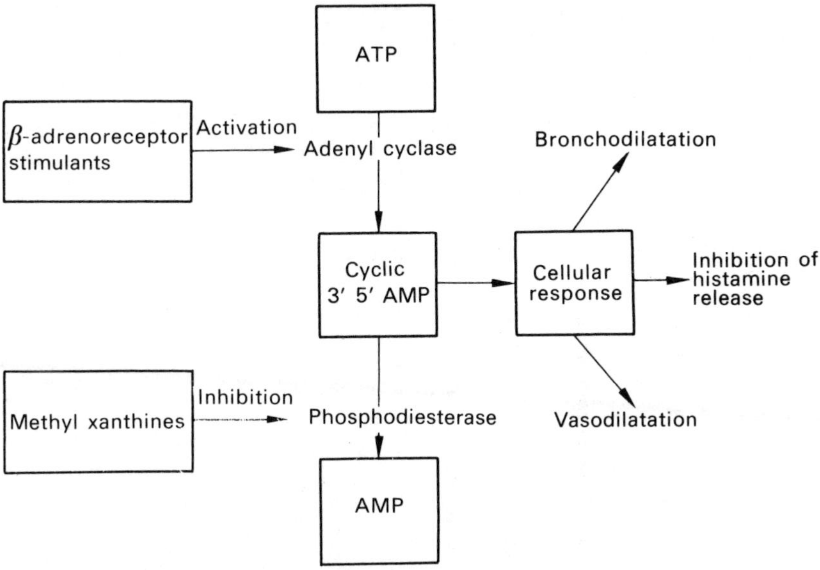

Fig. 9.2 The mode of action of beta adrenergic stimulants

In the airway, cyclic AMP inhibits the release of mast cell mediators as well as causing relaxation of bronchial smooth muscle. Until recently, the only useful effect of beta stimulants in asthma was thought to be on bronchial smooth muscle, but Assem and Schild[12] have shown that they may inhibit the release of spasmogens from mast cells sensitised by IgE or IgG antibodies.

As discussed earlier, Szentivanyi[13] has proposed the beta blockade theory of bronchial asthma. This suggests that asthmatic patients have a constitutional defect or deficiency of adenyl cyclase and, therefore, that their rate of formation of cyclic AMP is less than normal. Thus, in these individuals, beta adrenergic activity is inadequate to counteract the alpha adrenergic activity, which in any case is increased in asthmatic patients, resulting in an exaggerated contractile response to any agonistic stimuli. Recent work has been directed towards investigating the effects of alpha receptor blockade in asthmatic patients, using thymoxamine or phentolamine for this purpose. Results of these clinical investigations[14] sup-

Table 9.3 Adrenergic receptor stimulants

Bronchodilators	Routes of Administration			Pharmacological Effects			Side Effects	
	Oral	Inhaled	Injected	Alpha	$Beta_1$	$Beta_2$	Tachycardia	Skeletal Muscle Tremor
Adrenaline		•	•	•	•	•	•	•
Ephedrine	•			•	•	•	•	•
Isoprenaline, (Medihaler-Iso)		•			•	•	•	•
Orciprenaline (Alupent)	•	•			•	•	•	•
Isoetharine (Numotac)	•				•	•	•	•
Salbutamol (Ventolin)	•	•	•			•		•
Terbutaline (Bricanyl)	•	•	•			•		•
Rimiterol (Pulmadil)		•				•		

ported by biochemical studies suggest that alpha-receptor-blocking drugs in combination with beta-receptor stimulants may have a place in the management of asthma.

Clinical Studies

The currently available bronchodilator preparations, their pharmacological effects, routes of administration and side effects are shown in Table 9.3.

Oral preparations. The two most useful selective $beta_2$ adrenergic stimulants for childhood asthma are salbutamol and terbutaline. Several comparisons have been made in the treatment of bronchial asthma between these two oral preparations. Salbutamol is available in both 2 mg and 4 mg tablets, while terbutaline is available only as a 5 mg tablet. Legge and colleagues[15] found that, in adults, the bronchodilator effects of 5 mg of salbutamol were equivalent to those of 5 mg of terbutaline. Assessment of lung function showed a rise in forced expiratory volume in 1 second within half an hour of taking either drug. The response obtained was maximal between two and four hours and lasted for a minimum of five hours. A mean rise in heart rate of 8 beats/min was produced by each drug. Among the 12 patients studied, 4 experienced tremor following terbutaline and 5 following salbutamol. Interestingly, only 1 patient experienced tremor with both drugs; thus, because of individual variations in patient response, these drugs may provide useful alternatives.

Formgren[16] found that doses of 5 mg and 7·5 mg of terbutaline increased peak expiratory flow rate and forced expiratory volume in 1 second in a dose-dependent manner. Moreover, although no cardiovascular effects were seen with the 5 mg dose, a significant rise in heart rate was seen when the dose was increased to 7·5 mg. Kennedy and Simpson[17] showed that cardiovascular effects were present when doses of 8 mg of salbutamol were administered.

Leegaard and Fjulsrug[18] investigated 30 children in a double blind study. They showed that orally administered terbutaline (doses of 0·075 and 0·0375 mg/kg) produced marked bronchodilatation for a period of at least 5 hours without tachycardia.

Inhaled preparations. Pressurised aerosol preparations of salbutamol (100 μg per puff) and terbutaline (250 μg per puff) are available. Hambleton and Shinebourne,[19] in a double-blind placebo-controlled study of asthmatic children, showed that salbutamol (100 μg) produced similar bronchodilator activity (FEV_1) to that of isoprenaline (100 μg) but of longer duration. Inhalation of salbutamol (100 μg) and terbutaline by a group of asthmatic adults in a trial comparing one metered dose of each[20] showed that the bronchodilator responses were similar, although the duration of action was slightly longer with terbutaline. There were no clinically important cardiovascular or other unwanted effects from either drug in this study. It has also been shown that 200 μg of salbutamol gives a significantly greater response (FEV$_1$) than 250 μg of terbutaline.

Injected preparations. Terbutaline is available for subcutaneous use and, administered to adults (250 μg), caused the peak flow to rise at 15 minutes after injection.[21] The rise in maximal (40 per cent above base line) at 30 minutes and only a slight increase in heart rate was observed. Hansing and Kjellman[22] gave terbutaline subcutaneously to ten asthmatic children in a dose of 5 μg/kg, and this dose produced a useful increase in peak flow rate and no undesirable side effects were seen. Intravenous salbutamol is effective in producing bronchodilatation and has been well documented.[4] Salbutamol is at present undergoing clinical evaluation for use as a parenteral preparation and may replace adrenaline, which has both alpha and beta$_1$ effects, and become the treatment of choice. Some metabolic effects following intravenous[83] or oral[84] administration of salbutamol in adults have been recently described and need further evaluation. Terbutaline, salbutamol and orciprenaline, administered subcutaneously, have been compared in the treatment of asthmatic children admitted to hospital with acute attacks.[23] Each drug was given in doses of 1·75, 3·5 and 7·0 μg/kg at 8 hourly intervals on separate occasions. All drugs exhibited a marked effect on lung function, salbutamol and terbutaline being dose-dependent. Significant increases in peak expiratory flow rates were seen with these two drugs even at the lower dose levels.

Exercise-induced bronchoconstriction (EIB). The sympathomimetics adrenaline, ephedrine, isoprenaline, salbutamol and terbutaline have been shown to inhibit exercise-induced bronchoconstriction (EIB) if given before exercise.[24] When studying groups of asthmatic children who performed standardised treadmill running tests, Godfrey and Silverman[25] compared the effect of atropine, salbutamol and sodium cromoglycate. They found that salbutamol was the most effective in preventing EIB (Fig. 9.3).

In another study the protective effects of standard doses of several potential inhibitors of EIB were assessed.[26] It was found that salbutamol by aerosol or mouth was more effective than choline theophyllinate given orally, atropine methonitrate or sodium cromoglycate by inhalation. Fifteen asthmatic children were studied: EIB was blocked by atropine in 4 out of 7 subjects, by sodium cromoglycate in 12 out of 15, by choline theophyllinate also in 12, and by salbutamol in all 15 children.

II Sodium Cromoglycate

Sodium cromoglycate was first synthesised in 1965. It resulted from an in-

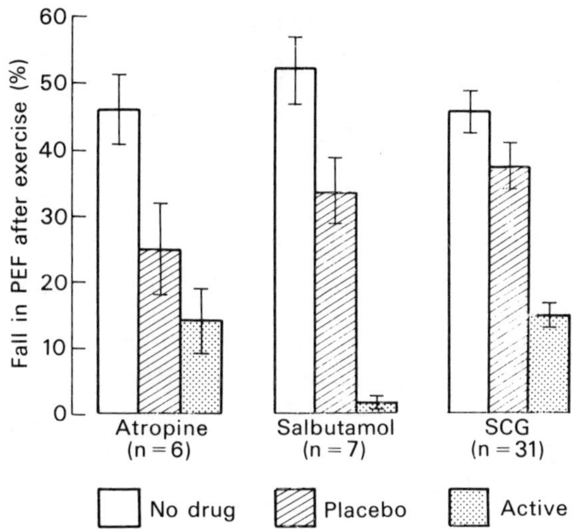

Fig. 9.3 The effect of atropine, salbutamol and sodium cromoglycate (SCG) compared with placebos on exercise-induced bronchoconstriction: the number of subjects studied is indicated for each drug. (*From* Godfrey and Silverman, 1973)

vestigation into the biological properties of synthetic analogues of khellin (Fig. 9.4), a naturally occurring cromone derivative obtained from the seeds of an eastern Mediterranean plant Ammi Visnaga. Khellin possesses the property of relaxing smooth muscle and was used in the treatment of colic, but because of its unpleasant side effects, nausea and vomiting, was never widely accepted. As the result of an effort to improve the ability of khellin to relax smooth muscle and, at the same time, to eliminate its undesirable side-effects, sodium cromoglycate was discovered.

Sodium cromoglycate is a new type of anti-asthmatic drug. It does not possess conventional anti-inflammatory properties, or corticosteroid-like effects, it is not a bronchodilator, and it is not a pharmacological antagonist of the mediators of tissue reaction such as histamine and slow reacting substance of anaphylaxis (SRS–A). It is thought to act by stabilising mast cell membranes, thereby inhibiting the release of pharmacological mediators when cells are triggered. It was found to be effective in sensitised individuals by reducing the asthmatic response to inhaled antigen, this protective effect lasting for several hours after administration.[27,28] Since its introduction into medicine in 1967, sodium cromoglycate has been the subject of many papers and review articles.[29,30]

Administration. Sodium cromoglycate is supplied in capsules containing 20 mg of the drug dispersed with 20 mg of lactose. It is administered from a specially designed inhaler (spinhaler) which spins and vibrates the

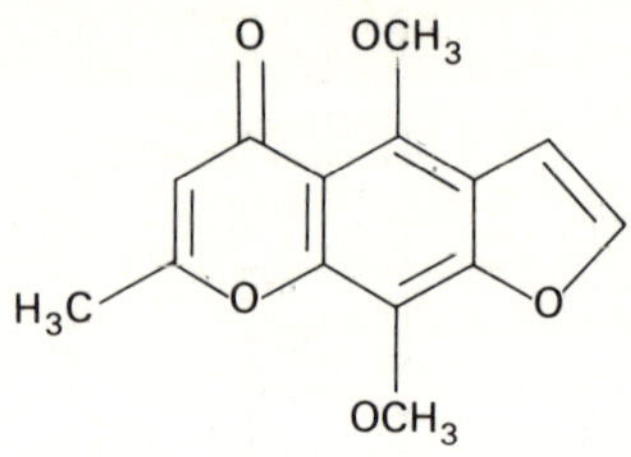

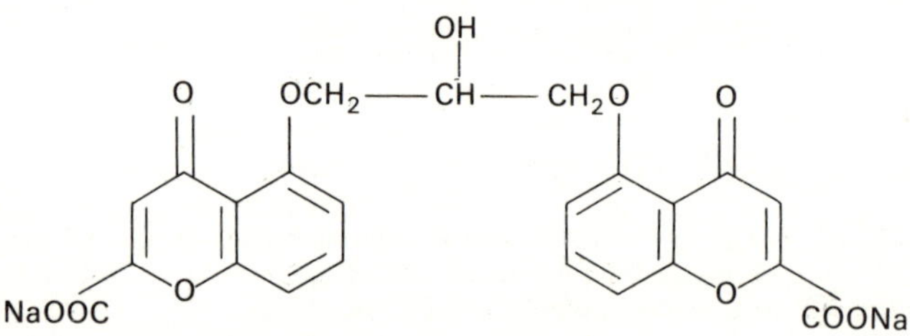

Fig. 9.4 The structures of khellin and sodium cromoglycate

capsule when the patient inspires, enabling the drug to be inhaled into the lungs as a powder. Occasionally, patients may experience cough and/or bronchospasm following inhalation of this powder and a preparation is available which contains as well as 20 mg of sodium cromoglycate, 100 μg of isoprenaline; the latter is present to counteract any transient bronchospasm. Because of the immediate relief of bronchoconstriction that patients obtain on using this combined preparation, ensuring its use prophylactically has often proved difficult. Although many trials published before 1970 were carried out using this combination it has been shown that the added isoprenaline gives little added therapeutic advantage,[31] and it is therefore preferable to prescribe plain sodium cromoglycate. If bronchospasm results from inhalation of the powder, the prior administration of a selective bronchodilator such as salbutamol, will often prevent this occurring and may enable more sodium cromoglycate to reach the airways.

Pharmacokinetics

The absorption metabolism and excretion of sodium cromoglycate has been investigated in asthmatic patients.[32] Less than 1 per cent of this compound is absorbed when given orally and, thus, it is completely ineffective by this route. Following inhalation, less than 5 per cent of the dose reaches the lungs; this small amount is absorbed rapidly and eliminated unchanged in the urine and bile without giving rise to any side effects. The majority of the dose, being deposited in the oropharynx, is swallowed and, not being absorbed, is excreted unchanged in the faeces. The amount that actually reaches the respiratory tract is dependent to some extent on the degree of airways obstruction present since, in patients with low inspiratory flow rates, less drug will be inhaled into the lungs. Maximum plasma levels of 9 ng/ml are obtained in asthmatic patients within 15 minutes of inhalation, and the plasma half-life is approximately 90 minutes.[32] Such rapid clearance of sodium cromoglycate from the plasma results in very little drug remaining after four hours. There appears to be no accumulation of the drug in the body and no toxic effects have been reported.

Mode of action. The principal mode of action of sodium cromoglycate in asthma is believed to involve the temporary stabilisation of the mast cell membranes (Fig 9.5). This action is thought to prevent the degranulation

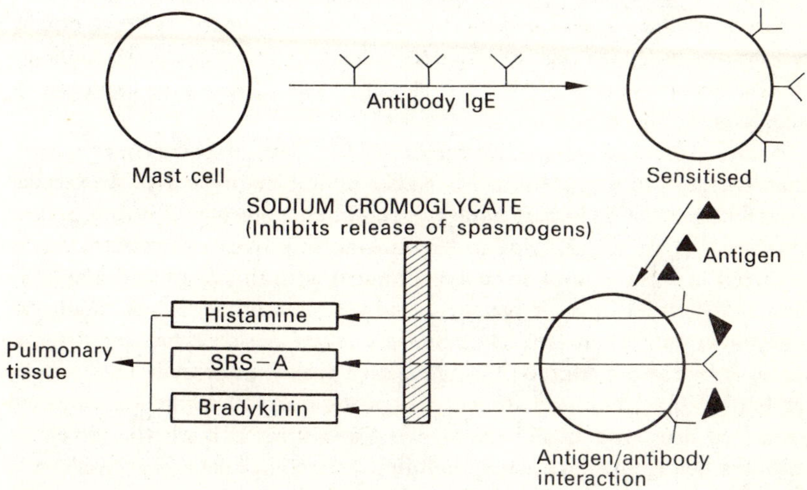

Fig. 9.5 The mode of action of sodium cromoglycate

of the cells and the subsequent release of the mediators of the type I immediate hypersensitivity reaction. Sodium cromoglycate can protect the mast cells from the effect both of immunological agents (antigen-antibody type) and non-immunological agents (such as phospholipase A, compound 48/80 and some surface active agents) and of exercise-induced bronchoconstriction. However, inhibition of degranulation, occurs only if sodium cromoglycate is present before the degranulation stimulus is received. This means that it is a prophylactic agent and has no direct effect on the interaction of antigen with antibody on the surface of sensitised mast cells.

Sodium cromoglycate also inhibits bronchoconstriction induced in man by alpha adrenoreceptor stimulation in the presence of beta blockade. A reduction in the degree of hypersensitivity to histamine has also been observed in some patients after prolonged administration. These observations raise the possibility that the drug may interact with adrenergic mechanisms and have a direct action on bronchial smooth muscle.

Bronchial challenge. The immediate type I asthmatic reaction to antigen challenge is effectively inhibited by pretreatment with sodium cromoglycate in the experimental situation.[33] The drug has the same effect in clinical practice when used prophylactically for the control of pollen-induced asthma. In addition, sodium cromoglycate has been shown to inhibit the development of the type III delayed reaction.[33] This late reaction, which may be accompanied by fever and leucocytosis, is poorly reversible by bronchodilators, although it is inhibited by corticosteroids which do not protect against type I reaction. However, sodium cromoglycate is unable to reverse bronchospasm when it has already occurred following exposure to allergens.

Exercise-induced bronchoconstriction (EIB). Several studies have shown that sodium cromoglycate can partially inhibit or prevent post-exercise bronchoconstriction in both adults and children if given a short time before exercise.[24] This effect helps to explain the improved exercise tolerance reported in some asthmatic children treated with this drug, and may also be a contributory factor in producing subjective improvement in childhood asthma without a concomitant increase in lung function as measured in the clinic or by the patient monitoring his own peak expiratory flow rate daily at home. Silverman and Andrea,[34] investigating 10 asthmatic children, found the drug was equally effective in diminishing EIB whether given 20 minutes before or immediately before exercise challenge. However, very little effect was seen with sodium cromoglycate when it was compared with placebo and administered at the end of the six-minutes exercise test. It has also been shown, in a group of asthmatic children, that the protective effect of this drug in EIB persists for only about four hours although it may give partial protection for up to six hours.[35] This time sequence agrees with the results obtained by Walker and colleagues[32] who measured plasma levels of sodium cromoglycate and found that these were maintained for about four hours only. Because of the limited duration of its maximal protective effect in patients who respond to this therapy a booster dose of the drug must be given within one hour of their anticipated exercise.

Clinical Evaluation

A major difficulty in evaluating any therapeutic regimen in asthma stems from the variable nature of the disease. Thereore, in order to make a valid comparison between two periods, frequent records of both subjective and objective data must be kept, particularly if a prophylactic therapy is being evaluated. The principal ways of evaluating the effect of treatment on the asthmatic state include: clinical examination, recording of symptoms on a

Card code H 3 0 1 0 5 _ _ Patient No. _ _ _ _

Card Number 1

Code	Item	Description	Score	1	2	3	4
01	Treatment Classification Code						
02	NIGHT	Good night Slept well but slightly wheezy Woken × 2 – 3 because of wheeze Bad night, awake most of time	0 1 2 3				
03	WHEEZE	None Little Moderately bad Severe	0 1 2 3				
04	ACTIVITY	Quite normal Can run short distance Limited to walking Off work/school or indoors } due to chest symptoms	0 1 2 3				
05	COUGH	None Occasional Frequent	0 1 2				
06	SPUTUM Add 'Y' if yellow	None Less than 3 tsps = a little More than 3 tsps = lot	0 1 2				
07	FLOW METER READING	Before breakfast dose of aerosal					
08		Before bedtime dose of aerosol					
9	NEW AEROSOL	New aerosol – Number of puffs in 24 hrs					
10	ADDI–TIONAL DRUGS	Bronchodilator – Number of puffs in 24 hrs Name:					
11		Intal Capsules – Number in 24 hrs					
12		Quantity others					
	COMMENTS – (Only if there is anything unusual to report) e.g. a cold						

Fig. 9.6 Symptom score card adapted from that originally described by Connolly and Godfrey, 1970

daily symptom score card (Fig 9.6), physiological measurements such as spirometry and peak expiratory flow rate measured periodically or daily, and the requirement for medication in addition to the drug under test.

In the management of children, a record of the number of days off school and the degree of restriction of exercise as evidenced by their ability to play games compared with other children can provide a useful means of assessing their asthmatic condition and the results of therapy.

Patient Selection

Prophylactic sodium cromoglycate is of considerable benefit to a few patients and of some benefit to many. In general, children with a strong evidence of allergy, a high Jones lability index, and for whom sodium cromoglycate produces a significant reduction in post-exercise airways obstruction, respond favourably to this drug more often than do those patients not exhibiting such features. Although there is a tendency towards a better response in patients with evidence of atopy, the apparent absence of allergic aetiology does not always preclude a favourable response. Children who are relatively free from symptoms between attacks of asthma often respond well to this drug, and there is a tendency for those with severe asthma to derive less benefit from sodium cromoglycate than those with mild or moderate symptoms.[36].

Adult Studies

Many short-term studies have demonstrated the superiority of sodium cromoglycate over placebo in patients with asthma of varying aetiology and severity. Although most of these studies have relied largely on the subjective assessment of therapeutic efficacy, about half have included an assessment of respiratory function. The results of a short-term double-blind trial in 252 patients[37] indicated a favourable response to sodium cromoglycate when compared with placebo in respect of symptom scores, physicians' evaluation, patient preference, and the need for oral bronchodilators. Statistically, pulmonary function was not significantly improved. Improvement in subjective criteria without a corresponding improvement in lung function has been noted in many other short-term studies and may have resulted, in part, from the simultaneous reduction of concomitant medication.

Satisfactory clinical evidence for the success of sodium cromoglycate has been established in the previously mentioned long-term controlled trial conducted at the Brompton Hospital.[31] In this study four comparable groups of patients with severe asthma were investigated for a period of 12 months. The patients were selected only if treatment with the usual therapeutic measures (with the exception of corticosteroids) was ineffective. They were randomly allocated to sodium cromoglycate, to sodium cromoglycate plus isoprenaline, to isoprenaline, or to placebo. The allocated treatment was regarded as failed if there were uncontrolled acute attacks or inadequate general control of the asthma requiring the deliberate addition of sodium cromoglycate or corticosteroids to the treatment.

Measurements of lung function were not made daily but forced expiratory volumes in one second were recorded during each patient's monthly visit to the clinic. Those patients who responded to their allocated treatment and, thus, continued on it showed statistically significant improvement in lung function at 24 and 52 weeks. At the end of the year's treatment there were only 5 failures out of 15 patients receiving sodium cromoglycate alone, and 4 failures among the 20 patients receiving sodium cromoglycate and isoprenaline. In contrast, there were 15 failures out of the 20 patients receiving only isoprenaline, and 16 out of the 19 patients receiving placebo. However, the possibility of a response to placebo, even after prolonged treatment, was clearly illustrated by this study. Sixteen weeks after beginning the trial 40 per cent of patients were adequately controlled with placebo plus standardised routine medication in spite of the fact that they had not been controlled by this regimen before the trial began.

This and other studies have shown that more than half of adult asthmatic patients show some degree of subjective improvement during long-term therapy with sodium cromoglycate. Thus, it is appropriate that all asthmatic patients be given a trial period of sodium cromoglycate therapy.

Studies in Children

There have been many short and long-term studies carried out in children.[30] The symptom scores monitored have shown some degree of improvement during therapy with sodium cromoglycate in 70 to 80 per cent of children investigated.

Collins-Williams and colleagues investigated 63 children with severe allergic asthma and found that the number of attacks, breathlessness, cough and times awakened at night lessened to a significant degree ($p < 0{\cdot}05$) during sodium cromoglycate therapy.[38] Several short-term studies in which the requirements for aerosol bronchodilators were recorded during periods of treatment have shown a significant reduction in their use during sodium cromoglycate therapy.[30]

The therapeutic efficacy of sodium cromoglycate was assessed in 27 children over a period of one year.[39] Absence from school and the number of hospital admissions were recorded and compared with data during one year when the children did not receive this therapy. Seventy four per cent of the children improved clinically while under treatment, and school absences showed a reduction of about 50 per cent. In two long-term open studies,[40,41] treatment with sodium cromoglycate was found to produce improvement in the ability to exercise, reduction in the frequency of asthma attacks, school absenteeism and admissions to hospital, improvement in nocturnal symptoms and decreased requirements for concomitant medication. However, because spontaneous improvement in the clinical condition of asthmatic children may occur in the course of a year, long-term studies of anti-asthmatic therapy must be controlled by the use of a standard drug or placebo.

There have been two long-term controlled double-blind studies of sodium cromoglycate in childhood asthma: one was a within-patient study lasting for 24 weeks[42] and the other was a between-patient trial continuing for one year.[43] In the first study, clinical evidence of improvement was seen in 14 out of 22 children with chronic asthma.[42] The patients had received either sodium cromoglycate or placebo for 12 weeks and then the alternative preparation for the remaining period. Lung function, measured at intervals of four weeks, improved significantly during active treatment.

In the second study,[43] 53 children with severe perennial asthma were divided into two groups and received treatment with either sodium cromoglycate plus isoprenaline or isoprenaline alone. At the end of one year, 71 per cent of the sodium cromoglycate group were well controlled compared with only 24 per cent of the isoprenaline group. By two of the methods of measuring lung function (forced expiratory volume in one second and peak expiratory flow rate) carried out at monthly intervals in the clinic, there were no differences between the two groups, although the forced vital capacity was significantly improved for those on sodium cromoglycate. However, in the measurements of peak expiratory flow rate made twice daily there was a highly significant improvement in the sodium cromoglycate group as compared with the group receiving only isoprenaline ($p < 0 \cdot 01$). This illustrates the need to monitor lung function frequently. In these groups 19 patients were investigated for exercise-induced bronchoconstriction: 8 out of 10 patients who benefited were on sodium cromoglycate compared with only 3 out of 9 patients who were not, and this was statistically significant ($p < 0 \cdot 05$).

Silverman and his colleagues could not detect any clear association between the duration and severity of asthma and the subsequent response to sodium cromoglycate. Jones and Blackhall[44] showed that the best clinical response was in those patients with a high lability index. They found that improvement occurred in 60 per cent of patients with normal lung function and in whom bronchial lability exceeded 30 per cent whereas only 25 per cent of those with a variable lability index and an abnormal forced expiratory volume in one second improved. Labile asthmatics have clear-cut attacks of asthma, with normal or near-normal respiratory function in between, while patients with variable lability have severe asthma with persistent symptoms and frequent attacks.

Corticosteroid-dependent Patients

Although many short-term studies have reported that the maintenance dosage of corticosteroids can be reduced or withdrawn during sodium cromoglycate therapy, long-term trials are necessary to determine the extent of any lasting reduction of systemic steroid requirements. The possibility of reducing maintenance corticosteroids varies greatly between individuals because of the widely differing initial dosages, duration of treatment, and different criteria for successful reduction. However, the important point is that any reduction of systemic steroids should be attempted only when the patient's asthma is well controlled on the usual dose. Special care must be taken after steroid withdrawal until the hypothalamic-pituitary-adrenal axis recovers fully. Important, also, is that in previously steroid-dependent patients severe exacerbations of asthma must be treated promptly with large doses of corticosteroids.

Chai and colleagues[45] adjusted corticosteroid dosage while maintaining each child in a similar clinical condition as before sodium cromoglycate therapy was started. This trial was a 12 week double-blind study followed by a 6 to 12 month observation period. By the addition of sodium cromoglycate a significant reduction in corticosteroid requirements, or a change from once or twice daily to alternate day therapy was possible in about half of all the children studied. During the follow-up period a further reduction (25 per cent) in corticosteroid requirement was achieved in 5 out of 13 patients for whom a reduction of less than 50 per cent had been possible during the double blind phase.

Some authors, although not monitoring lung function, have carefully compared corticosteroid requirements during sodium cromoglycate therapy with that during the corresponding months of a previous year. Engström and Kraepelien,[46] studying 44 children, reported corticosteroid requirements to be significantly lower during six months treatment with sodium cromoglycate than during the previous year, there being no significant difference between two control years.

Side Effects

The side effects of sodium cromoglycate most commonly reported have been irritation of throat and trachea.[30] However, these symptoms have generally been infrequent, mild and transient and have seldom necessitated the withdrawal of sodium cromoglycate. No changes in haemaglobin, white blood and eosinophil cells, blood urea, SGOT, SGPT and urinalysis have been noted.[43] A study conducted among a group of 82 children who had received therapeutic dosages of sodium cromoglycate for three years revealed no detectable radiological changes in the lungs, nor any evidence of renal, hepatic or haematological changes attributable to the use of this drug.[30] No reports have indicated that sodium cromoglycate has adverse effects on growth, or any direct effect on adrenal function.

III Steroid Aerosols

Corticosteroids are the most effective group of chemotherapeutic agents for the treatment of all types of asthma. They have been given systemically since their introduction into medicine in the early 1950s, but the risk of serious side effects that accompanies continuous administration has limited their use. However, for some patients there is no alternative therapy; adequate symptomatic relief cannot be obtained from bronchodilators or sodium cromoglycate.

Although the mode of action of glucocorticoids is not understood, there have been a number of suggested mechanisms that may have some relevance to their effectiveness in the treatment of reversible airways obstruction. The inflammatory response may be reduced and possible mechanisms includes—

1. A vascular effect on minute vessels and arterioles, the stabilisation of lysosomal membranes and the inhibition of the passage of leucocytes out of the microcirculation.
2. Inhibition of the mediators of inflammation, i.e. prostaglandins, kinins and histamine.
3. The sensitisation of beta adrenergic receptors to catecholamine stimulation and promotion of the formation of cyclic AMP.

The rationale of inhaled steroids. Corticosteroids were first given by inhalation to asthmatic patients because the hope was that a high local concentration in the lung might achieve therapeutic benefit while avoiding the undesirable side-effects associated with systemic administration. Although some corticosteroids given in this way (Table 9.4) have produced a certain

Table 9.4 Corticosteroids used by inhalation for asthma

1950	Cortisone
1951	Hydrocortisone
1958	Prednisolone
1963	Dexamethasone
1972	Beclomethasone dipropionate
1973	Betamethasone valerate

degree of success, the therapeutic response obtained with cortisone, hydrocortisone and prednisolone was disappointing.[47–49] Subsequent studies with dexamethasone phosphate[50] and, later, with dexamethasone isonicotinate given by inhalation resulted in a favourable response in a significant proportion of both adults and children, although this was often accompanied by adrenal suppression and hypercortism.[50,51] Therefore, the steroid aerosols investigated in the 1950s and 1960s seemed to offer very little advantage over the administration of these drugs systemically.

The introduction, in the 1970s, of beclomethasone dipropionate and betamethasone valerate (Fig. 9.7) was a significant advance in inhalation therapy. These two steroid aerosols have characteristics that make them highly effective in the treatment of reversible airways obstruction, while at the same time not affecting hypothalamic-pituitary-adrenal function at therapeutic doses.

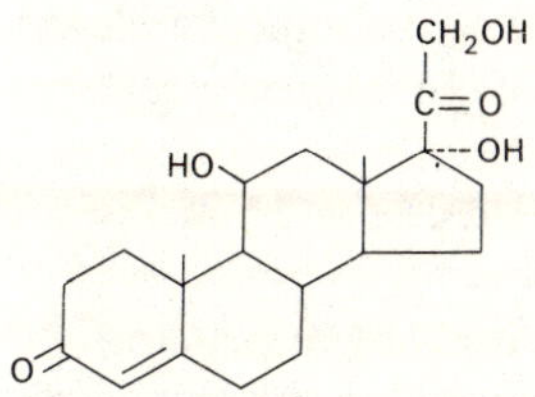

HYDROCORTISONE

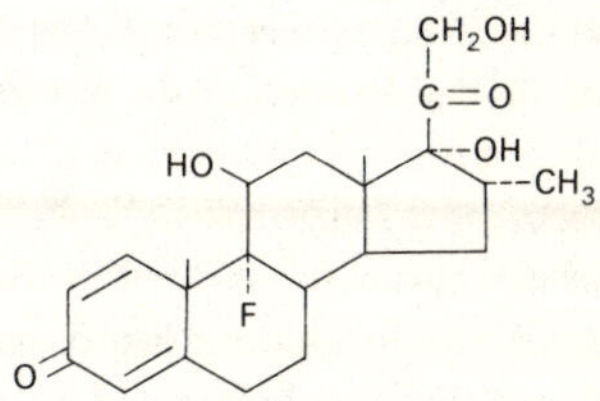

DEXAMETHASONE

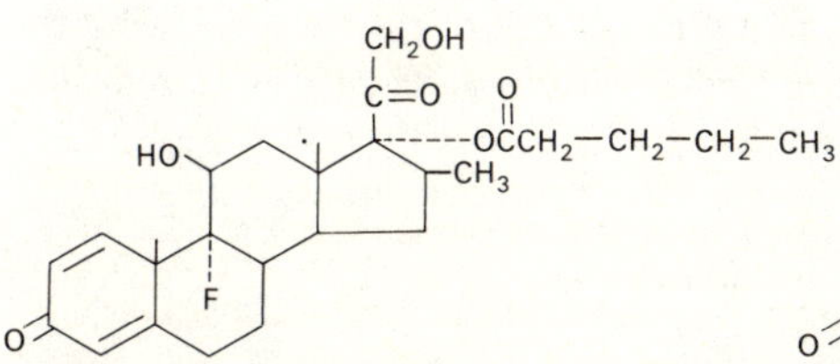

BETAMETHASONE VALERATE

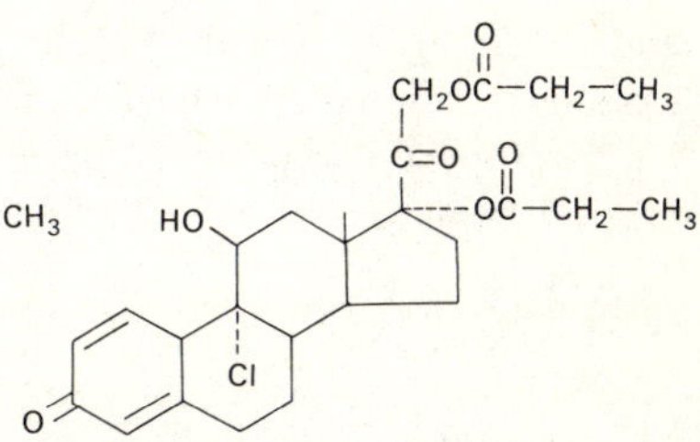

BECLOMETHASONE DIPROPIONATE

Fig. 9.7 The structures of some corticosteroids given by inhalation

The three currently available steroid aerosols for the treatment of asthma are dexamethasone isonicotinate*, beclomethasone diproprionate and betamethasone valerate. The dexamethasone isonicotinate aerosol delivers 125 μg per puff and its recommended dosage is one to two puffs five times a day (a total daily dose of 625–1250 μg, although up to 2,000 μg/day may be given). The beclomethasone dipropionate inhalers deliver

* Not available in Great Britain

50 μg per puff and the betamethasone valerate aerosol 100 μg per puff. The recommended daily dosage in children for each of these is 400 to 800 μg although doses of up to 1,600 μg/day may be required in some adults. It is important that having initiated therapy at the maximum recommended daily dose, this should be reduced to the minimum necessary adequately to control the patient's asthmatic symptoms. This may be as low as 100 μg twice daily in some children.

Aerosol deposition. Recent studies of the pharmacokinetics of inhaled drugs[9,32] have demonstrated that only a small amount of the dose inhaled from an aerosol, probably of the order of 10 per cent, actually reaches the lungs; the remainder (90 per cent) is deposited in the mouth and swallowed. Thus, an aerosol can be regarded as providing two doses: one that is deposited in the lungs (a topical dose) and one that reaches the gastrointestinal tract (an oral dose). For a steroid aerosol to have any advantage over systemic therapy, the small dose reaching the lungs must produce a therapeutic response while the combined activity of the topical and oral dose must be less than that that will suppress the hypothalamic-pituitary-adrenal axis.

Topical and systemic activity. The fact that inhalation is an inefficient method of depositing a drug in the lungs may partly explain the absence of any advantage in using steroids such as dexamethasone by this route. The ideal corticosteroid for use by aerosol has been postulated as having a high topical activity but a week systemic effect. In 1962, a reliable method of predicting topical anti-inflammatory activity was developed by McKenzie and Stoughton based on the measurement of the blanching or vasoconstriction corticosteroids cause in intact skin.[52] Results showing the relative topical and systemic potencies of various corticosteroids and their inhaled doses are given in Table 9.5.

Table 9.5

Corticosteroid	*Topical Activity	†Systemic Activity(mg)	Inhaled Dose(mg)
Cortisone	0	25	50
Hydrocortisone	<1	30	15–45
Prednisolone	<1	10	1‡
Betamethasone	<1	1	—
Dexamethasone isonicotinate	1·5	1	0·5–2·0
Betamethasone valerate	360	10	0·4–1·6
Beclomethasone dipropionate	500	10	0·4–1·0

* Measured by the vasoconstrictor test on human skin (arbitary scale)
† Approximate oral adrenal-suppressing dose in man
‡ No therapeutic benefit from this low dose

The earlier corticosteroids that were given by inhalation have poor topical anti-inflammatory activity, dexamethasone and betamethasone being little better than prednisolone and hydrocortisone in this respect. The systemic dose at which a steroid causes adrenal suppression seems to parallel its systemic anti-inflammatory activity in man and by this criterion dexamethasone and betamethasone are potent steroids when administered orally. Thus, none of these steroids fulfils the necessary requirements for being successful when given by inhalation and, as Table 9.5 shows, the effective inhaled dose was similar to that used systemically.

Betamethasone valerate and beclomethasone dipropionate given orally are about ten times weaker in their systemic activity than betamethasone, while topically they are very potent. Thus, there is a dissociation of topical from systemic effect with betamethasone valerate and beclomethasone dipropionate and they were selected as steroids likely to be useful by inhalation in asthma.

Human pharmacology. Betamethasone valerate, beclomethasone dipropionate and dexamethasone isonicotinate have been given by inhalation to healthy human adult volunteers.[53] Inhaled doses of between 4 and 8 mg/day of betamethasone valerate and beclomethasone dipropionate (ten times the normal therapeutic dose) were found to cause a significant change (30 to 50 per cent reduction) in the morning plasma cortisol levels (Fig. 9.8). Dexamethasone isonicotinate was, however, approximately five times as potent in its suppressing potential, causing significant depression of endogenous plasma cortisol at between 500 to 1000 μg/day (doses well within the therapeutic range).

Daily doses of 1600 μg of betamethasone valerate by inhalation taken for a week were found not to have any effect on morning plasma cortisol or, in the response, to short tetracosactrin or insulin stress tests.[54] Daily doses of 1,000 μg of beclomethasone dipropionate were similarly without effect on plasma corticosteroid or urinary oxogenic steroid levels in normal healthy adults.[55] By contrast, the inhalation of 1,250 μg/day of dexamethasone isonicotinate has a marked effect on hypothalamic-pituitary-adrenal function. The difference in the human pharmacology of dexamethasone isonicotinate and that of betamethasone valerate and beclomethasone dipropionate is reflected in clinical observations.

Clinical studies in adults. Beclomethasone dipropionate and betamethasone valerate were first investigated with promising results in steroid-dependent adult patients. Those selected had moderate to severe asthma and had been on continuous oral corticosteroid therapy for many years and several attempts at withdrawal of systemic steroids had resulted in the return of severe asthmatic symptoms. In general, they were treated with inhaled steroids if systemic steroid side-effects had been causing concern either to the patient or to the clinician responsible. Most patients were in a reasonably stable state when treatment with steroid aerosols (400 to 800 μg/day) was begun.

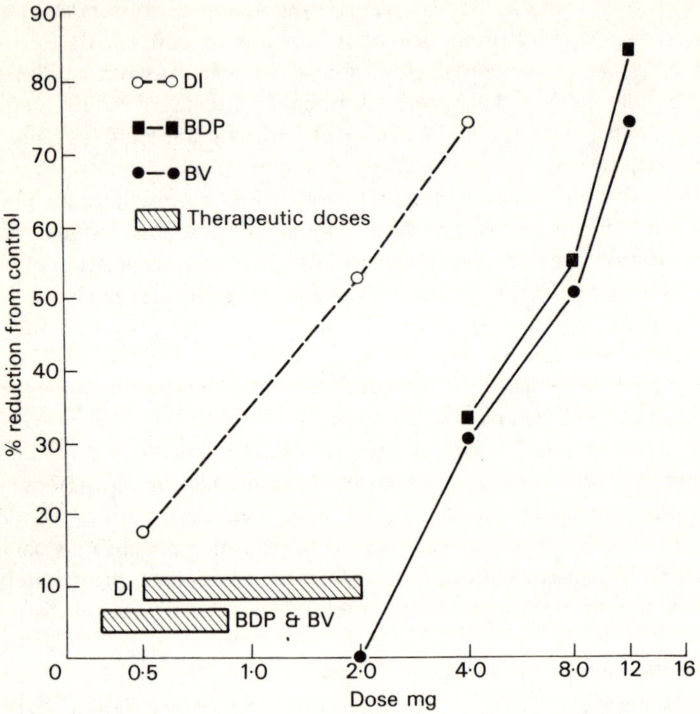

Fig. 9.8 Dose response curves showing effect of corticosteroids on plasma cortisol levels. (*From* Sparkes, 1974)

Recent surveys[56,57,81] report that about 70 per cent of patients dependent on oral corticosteroids alone, or on ACTH with or without additional oral corticosteroid therapy can be transferred to inhaled beclomethasone dipropionate or betamethasone valerate treatment. Better results are often obtained in children, whose asthma is more readily reversible, than with older patients who may have bronchial mucus or fixed airways obstruction.

The lack of systemic side-effects of beclomethasone dipropionate and betamethasone valerate aerosols has led to their investigation in adults for whom oral steroiods have not been used. Studies have included patients with chronic asthma who were being considered for oral steroid treatment or who may have received intermittent courses of systemic steroids previously, and patients poorly maintained on bronchodilators and/or sodium cromoglycate.

As these steroid aerosols are prophylactic they should be considered for patients requiring regular treatment only, not for those who have only occasional attacks of asthma.

Clinical Studies in Children

Bronchial asthma in childhood differs in some ways from that seen in adults. About half of adult patients will have some evidence of allergy, whereas more than 90 per cent of children having asthmatic symptoms will be atopic subjects and give positive skin tests to common allergens.[58] Because of these allergic factors, and because airways obstruction in children tends to be readily reversible, childhood asthma is particularly responsive to sodium cromoglycate and steroid treatment. However, systemic steroids have the particular disadvantage in children of adversely affecting growth. The advent of betamethasone valerate and beclomethasone dipropionate aerosols means that the therapeutic benefit of systemic steroids may be obtained while avoiding growth retardation, impaired adrenal function and cushingoid features.

Steroid-dependent children. Several studies of the use of beclomethasone dipropionate aerosols have been conducted in steroid-dependent children. Twenty-one children receiving oral corticosteroid therapy in addition to sodium cromoglycate were treated with inhaled beclomethasone dipropionate.[59] All improved or maintained their asthma status over a period of four months and stopped their regular systemic steroids, although four had to revert to their original therapy. Godfrey and König[60] studied 18 children taking systemic steriods and successfully weaned them from these, substituting inhaled steroids generally within two months. All but one of the children were satisfactorily controlled on this regimen although 15 needed short courses of oral steroids at times of severe exacerbations. The aerosol dosage varied between 100 and 800 μg/day according to the clinical response obtained. There was no evidence of adrenal suppression after treatment with beclomethasone dipropionate for one year. In another study,[61] 15 out of 16 children dependent on oral corticosteroid or corticotrophin for up to eleven years were successfully transferred to beclomethasone dipropionate by inhalation.

Systemic steroid withdrawal. The substitution of inhaled for systemic steroids should be attempted only under careful clinical and spirometric control and when the patient's asthma is stable. Common withdrawal effects include headache, nausea, vomiting, anorexia, backache and depression. Emotional instability may occasionally last for a week or longer, and malaise, muscle and joint pain may last for several months. Specific treatment may be needed for unmasked allergic rhinitis and eczema. The emergence of these sysmptoms is indirect evidence that the inhaled steroids are not having systemic effects, and patients need encouragement and support during the withdrawal of systemic steroids. Indirect evidence of the purely local activity of the steroids is also provided by the regression of cushingoid features,[62] relief of dyspepsia, increase in blood eosinophilia, reduction in insulin requirements in diabetic patients, and resumption of a normal growth pattern in children.[63]

The desirability of slow withdrawal of oral steroids when transferring patients to steroid aerosols is emphasised by most physicians, as there is a risk of adrenal failure until hypothalamic-pituitary-adrenal function has fully recovered. Grant[64] feels that any reduction should be at the rate of 1 mg of prednisolone a day at monthly intervals, whereas Clark[65] advocates a more rapid transfer when possible, i.e. within a few weeks for patients taking 10 mg a day of prednisolone. The safe rate of withdrawal will depend on the level and previous duration of oral steroid dosage. What must be emphasised is that steroid-dependent patients may be at risk for up to one year after withdrawal of systemic corticosteroids. Patients recently weaned off oral steroids are in a precarious condition in the event of trauma, stress or infection, and they should be instructed to resume oral steroids immediately if there is any doubt that full hypothalamic-pituitary-adrenal responsiveness may not have returned. A supply of steroid tablets and warning cards should be given to all patients, and severe exacerbations of asthma should be treated promptly and vigorously with systemic steroids.

Children not receiving systemic steroids. Several studies have been carried out with betamethasone valerate aerosol in children. Frears and colleagues, in a double blind cross-over trial, compared two placebo periods with two periods of betamethasone valerate treatment alternating at monthly intervals (Fig. 9.9) in 20 severely asthmatic children.[66] The average of the twice-daily peak expiratory flow rates was increased in every child during the activity-treated months compared with the placebo months, each child having fewer symptoms while using a steroid aerosol, the average reduction for the group being 71 per cent. Less additional medication for asthma was required during months of the active treatment and the observed clinical response to therapy was dramatic in over half the children.

Evidence that inhaled steroids are effective because of local rather than systemic action was provided by Frears and colleagues.[67] They conducted a double blind study in 10 asthmatic children, comparing the clinical effect of one month's treatment of oral betamethasone valerate (1 mg/day) with one month of inhaled drug (800 μg/day). Results showed that on inhaled, compared with oral, steroids nine subjects had fewer symptoms, a higher mean twice daily peak expiratory flow rate and lower bronchodilator requirements, and all these changes were statistically significant. Thus, orally administered betamethasone valerate has no appreciable clinical effect on childhood asthma at the daily dose used but is highly effective by inhalation.

Taylor and Norman studied a group of severely asthmatic children who were not steroid-dependent by comparing betamethasone valerate aerosol with placebo.[68] A statistically significant improvement with the active drug

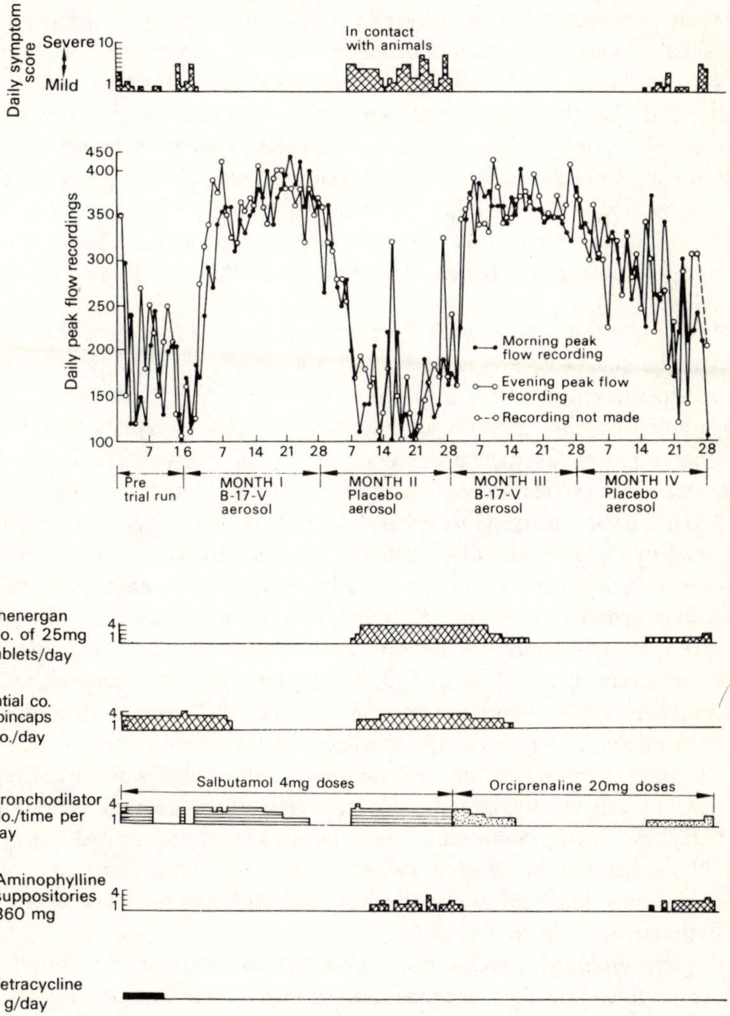

Fig. 9.9 A clinical comparison of betamethasone valerate and placebo in an asthmatic child, showing asthma symptom score, twice-daily peak flow readings and asthma therapy. (*From* Frears, Wilson and Friedman, 1973)

was shown by 17 of the 18 children as assessed by diary score cards, morning and evening peak flow rates, salbutamol aerosol usage, chest examination, height and weight gain, and monthly respiratory function tests.

Betamethasone valerate and sodium cromoglycate. Inhaled betamethasone valerate has been compared with sodium cromoglycate in childhood asthma.[69] Forty children were studied and both these drugs were found to be effective in reducing the mean total weekly asthmatic symptom score from that recorded during a placebo period. In general, the patients and physicians preferred betamethasone valerate to treatment with sodium cromoglycate ($p < 0{\cdot}05$). The peak expiratory flow rates measured in the clinic, and also those measured twice daily at home were significantly in favour of the inhaled steroid ($p < 0{\cdot}001$). Studies with betamethasone valerate in 10 children with chronic perennial asthma[70] who had symptoms that were not well-controlled on sodium cromoglycate alone, confirmed that in these cases it was clinically superior to sodium cromoglycate although no additional benefit was seen when the two drugs were given together.

Adrenal function and growth. The long-term maintenance of children on betamethasone valerate aerosol and its effect on the hypothalamic-pituitary-adrenal axis has also been studied.[71] More than fifty children maintained on this therapy for between one and two years had normal adrenal function as measured by monthly plasma cortisol levels. The response to short tetracosactrin tests was investigated in some children and found to be normal. Cortisol and ACTH release in response to insulin-induced hypoglycaemia was normal in 10 children receiving this therapy for 9 months and they had not previously been given systemic steroids.[71] In addition, growth rates and growth hormone levels were monitored in children receiving inhaled betamethasone valerate. The conclusion was that long-term therapy (200 to 800 μg a day) is unlikely to cause significant suppression of the hypothalamic-pituitrary-adrenal axis and that it allows growth to continue normally in children.

Kuzemko[63] has show that oral corticosteroids, in doses usually accepted as safe (5 mg prednisolone/day), adversely affect growth rates before puberty. However, betamethasone valerate aerosol controlled the symptomes of asthma in those children when they were transferred from systemic steroids, and the steroid aerosol did not interfere with their growth pattern (Fig. 9.10).

Exercise-induced bronchoconstriction (EIB). Investigation of the effect of corticosteroids on the response to exercise in asthmatic subjects has produced conflicting results. Acute studies have shown that hydrocortisone is of no benefit and inhaled beclomethasone dipropionate caused improvement in only 3 out of 11 children studied.[72] However, after prolonged administration, Heimlich and colleagues demonstrated definite benefit in a group of 29 children given oral prednisolone (20 mg/day) for 3 days before exercise tests.[73] while other investigators using the same drug (12 to 40 mg/day) for one week demonstrated improvement in only 3 out of 9 patients. Similarly, the administration of beclomethasone dipropionate daily for one to four weeks showed improvement in only 1 out of 6 children studied.[72]

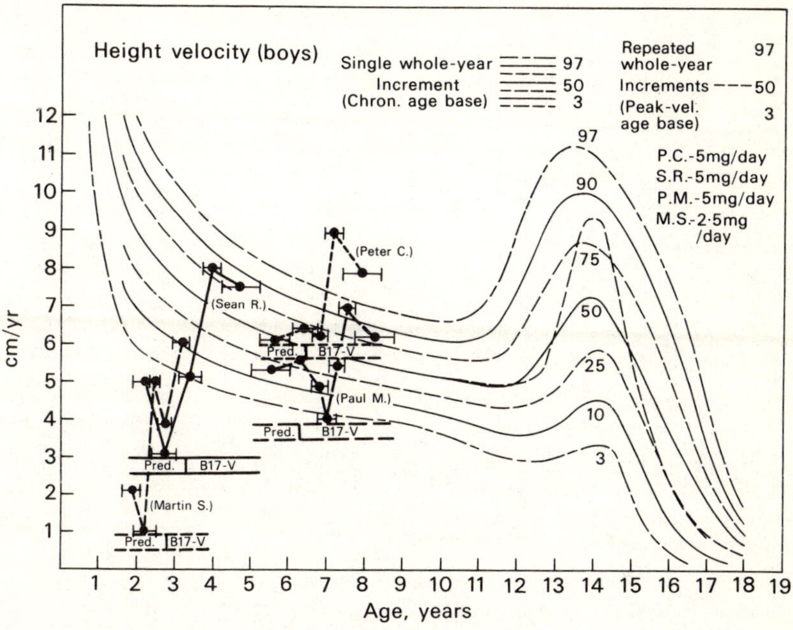

Fig. 9.10 Growth velocity in four pre-pubertal boys on oral corticosteroids (pred) and betamethasone valerate aerosol (B 17–V). (*From* Kuzemko, 1974)

A group of ten asthmatic children were studied and betamethasone valerate was not found to be effective in preventing EIB when given immediately before or 30 minutes before exercise, whereas salbutamol abolished EIB in these children.[74] However, long-term maintenance with betamethasone valerate reduced EIB in most children and withdrawal of this treatment led to its reappearance.

Side Effects

The possible side-effects of inhaled steroids that must be considered are depression of hypothalamic-pituitary-adrenal function, local effects on collagen synthesis, and increased incidence of infection. Evidence has

Table 9.6

Author	Steroid	Dose (μ/day)	Patients	No. in series	% symptomatic thrush	% asymptomatic thrush	Duration of follow-up (months)
1. Brown and Storey (1975)	BDP	400	Adults & Children	267	2	—	Up to 48
2. Grant (1975)	BDP	400	Adults	322	7	—	12
3. McAllen and Colleagues (1974)	BDP	400	Adults & Children	80	15	—	12
4. Milne and Crompton (1974)	BDP	400	Adults	177	6	—	6
5. Brown and Storey (1973)	BDP	400	Children	31	0	13	Up to 20
6. Friedman[79] (1975)	BV	200–800	Children	53	0	6	24
7. Godfrey and König (1974)	BDP	400	Children	24	0	0	2–24
8. Kuzemko[80] (1975)	BV	400	Children	100	0	0	12

already been presented that inhaled beclomethasone dipropionate and betamethasone valerate do not affect adrenal function at therapeutic doses.

Local effects. The suggestion has been made that atrophic changes in the bronchial mucosa may result from continuous treatment with inhaled steroid. This idea has arisen because of the atrophic effects occasionally seen when large amounts of topical steroid preparations are applied to a patient's skin for long periods. However, in terms of the amount of steroid per unit area, inhaling 800 μg of betamethasone valerate, of which probably only about 10 per cent is deposited in the lungs, could be compared with applying only 1 mg of betamethasone valerate cream to the whole body surface. Toxicity studies in dogs[75] given steroid aerosols over many months in doses high enough to render them grossly Cushingoid, produced no changes in any part of the respiratory tract from fauces to alveoli when these were examined at nine levels at post mortem. In addition, investigations among adults in Sweden[76] and Denmark,[77] have shown that lung tissue taken from patients treated with inhaled beclomethasone dipropionate for periods of six to twelve months at a dose level of 400 μg a day was similar to that seen in asthmatic patients who have not had this type of therapy.

Candidiasis. The only significant side-effect noted in adults receiving steroid aerosols is occasional transient hoarseness and localised colonisation of the mouth and throat with *Candida albicans*. Not all clinical investigators have reported candidiasis, and none has found it difficult to eradicate except in one or two cases, and treatment with either nystatin or amphotericin B proved successful.

Candida albicans may be isolated from about a third of the normal population. Milne and Crompton[78] took throat swabs from 936 patients who attended a respiratory diseases unit over a period of six months. Of these, 510 were being treated with a steroid inhaler, 143 with oral prednisolone, and 283 were not receiving any form of corticosteroid therapy. Candida species (predominantly, *Candida albicans*) were isolated from 41 per cent of swabs taken from patients receiving beclomethasone dipropionate compared with 30 per cent taken from the other patients.

The percentage of adult patients using steroid aerosols who have symptomatic candidiasis, clinical lesions and positive cultures appears to be about 8 per cent (Table 9.6). However, there is a wide variation in incidence reported in the literature. Brown and Storey[62] found a 2 per cent incidence in a series of 267 patients treated with beclomethasone dipropionate for up to four years. Grant[64] found symptomatic candidiasis in 21 out of 322 patients (7 per cent) while McAllen and colleagues[57] reported an incidence of 15 per cent. In one survey,[78] 6 per cent of the beclomethasone dipropionate patients had both symptoms and positive candida swabs. Because of the discomfort that this infection may cause and also because of the risk that it could spread further down the bronchial tree, therapy may have to be stopped in the troublesome or recurrent cases (less than 1 per cent). There has been no increased incidence of bacterial or viral infection in patients receiving inhaled steroids, and no cases of candida infection of the lung have been reported.

There is good evidence that the incidence of oral thrush is dose-related and is higher when 800 μg/day of the steroid aerosol is given than when the dose is 400 μg/day or less. However, the problem does not seem to occur to the same extent in children. Although asymptomatic candida (clinical lesions and positive swab cultures only) has been seen by some observers in a few patients (Table 9.6), no cases of symptomatic candida have been reported.

The conclusion is that betamethasone valerate and beclomethasone dipropionate given by inhalation are highly effective forms of therapy for the long-term prophylactic treatment of severe childhood asthma that does not respond to bronchodilators or sodium cromoglycate.

Further Suggested Reading

Asthma, Physiology, Immunopharmacology and Treatment (Ed. K. Austen and L. M. Lichtenstein). New York and London: Academic Press.

Bronchodilators (Paterson, G. W. and Spenfield, G. M.) Tubercle Supplement, *B.T.T.A. Review* (1974), **4,** 25.

Sodium cromoglycate (cromolyn sodium): a review of its mode of action, pharmacology, therapeutic efficacy and use (Brogden, R. N., Speight, T. M. and Avery, G. S.) *Drugs*, (1975), **7,** 164.

Betamethasone valerate aerosol in asthma. *Postgraduate Medical Journal*, (1974), **50,** Supplement 4.

Beclomethasone dipropionate aerosols (1975) *Postgraduate Medical Journal*, **51,** Supplement 4.

References

1. Ahlquist, R. P. (1948) A study of adrenotropic receptors. *American Journal of Physiology*, **153,** 586.
2. Lands, A. M., Arnold, A., McAuliff, J. P., Luduena, F. P. and Brown, T. G. (1967) Differentiation of receptor systems activated by sympathomimetic amines. *Nature*, **214,** 597.
3. Dollery, C. T. (1973) Symposium on isoproterenol therapy in asthma. *Annals of Allergy*, **31,** 25.
4. Paterson, J. W., Evans, R. J. and Prime, F. J. (1971) Selectivity of bronchodilator action of salbutamol in asthmatic patients. *British Journal of Diseases of the Chest*, **65,** 21.
5. Shenfield, G. M. and Paterson, J. W. (1973) Clinical assessment of bronchodilator drugs delivered by aerosol. *Thorax*, **28,** 124.
6. Paterson, J. W., Conolly, M. E., Davies, D. S. and Dollery, C. T. (1968) Isoprenaline resistance and the use of pressurised aerosols in asthma. *Lancet*, **2,** 426.
7. McEvoy, J. D. S., Vall-Spinosa, A. and Paterson, J. W. (1973) Assessment of orciprenaline and isoproterenol infusions in asthmatic patients. *American Review of Respiratory Diseases*, **108,** 490.

8. Jack, D. (1971) An introduction to salbutamol and other modern beta-adrenoreceptor stimulants. *Postgraduate Medical Journal*, **47,** (Supplement), p. 8.
9. Walker, S. R., Evans, M. E., Richards, A. J., Paterson, J. W. (1972) The clinical pharmacology of oral and inhaled salbutamol. *Clinical Pharmacology and Therapeutics*, **13,** 861.
10. Davies, D. S., George, C. F., Blackwell, E. W., Conolly, M. E. and Dollery, C. T. (1974) Metabolism of terbutaline in man and dog. *British Journal of Pharmacology*, **1,** 129.
11. Evans, M. E., Shenfield, G. M., Thomas, N, Walker, S. R. and Paterson, J. W. (1974) The pharmacokinetics of Rimiterol in man. *Xenobictica,* **4,** No 11, 681.
12. Assem, E. S. K. and Schild, H. O. (1969) Inhibition by sympathomimetic amines of histamine release by antigen in passively sensitized human lung. *Nature*, **224,** 1028.
13. Szentivanyi, A. (1968) The beta adrenergic theory of the atopic abnormality in bronchial asthma. *Journal of Allergy*, **42,** 203.
14. Patel, K. E. and Keer, J. W. (1975) Alpha-receptor-blocking drugs in bronchial asthma. *Lancet*, **1,** 348.
15. Legge, J. S., Gaddie, J., and Palmer, K. N. V. (1971) Comparison of two oral selective β_2 adrenergic stimulant drugs in bronchial asthma. *British Medical Journal*, **1,** 637.
16. Formgren, H. (1970) A clinical comparison of the effect of oral terbutaline and orciprenaline. *Scandinavian Journal of Respiratory Diseases,* **51,** 195.
17. Kennedy, M. C., and Simpson, W. T. (1969) Human pharmacological and clinical studies on salbutamol: a specific β adrenergic bronchodilator, *British Journal of Diseases of the Chest*, **63,** 165.
18. Leegaard, J. and Fjulsrug, S. (1973) Terbutaline in children with asthma. *Archives of Diseases in Childhood*, **48,** 229.
19. Hambleton, G. and Shinebourne, E. A. (1970) Evaluation of the effects of isoprenaline and salbutamol aerosols on airways obstruction and pulse rates of children with asthma. *Archives of Diseases in Childhood*, **45,** 766.
20. Freedman, B. J. (1972) Trail of a terbutaline aerosol in the treatment of asthma and a comparison of its effects with those of a salbutamol aerosol. *British Journal of Diseases of the Chest*, **66,** 222.
21. Arnes, B, Berteer, A, Karleford, T., *et al.* (1975) Bronchodilator effect of a new sympathomimetic β-receptor stimulating agent, terbutaline, given subcutaneously to asthmatic patients. *Acta Medical Scandinavian Supplement*, **512,** 41.
22. Hansing, B. and Kjellman, B. (1972) The effect of a new sympathomimetic β-receptor stimulating agent, terbutaline, given subcutaneously to asthmatic children. *Acta Allergologica*, **27,** 130.
23. Koivikko, A. (1974) A comparison of the effects of subcutaneous orciprenaline, salbutamol and terbutaline in asthmatic children. *Annals of Clinical Research*, **6,** 99.
24. Anderson, S. D., Silverman, M., König, P. and Godfrey, S. (1975) Exercise-induced asthma. *British Journal of Diseases of the Chest*, **69,** 1.
25. Godfrey, S. and Silverman, M. (1973) Demonstration of placebo response in asthma by means of exercise testing. *Journal of Psychosomatic Research,* **17,** 293.
26. Godfrey, S. and König, P. (1974) A comparison of the effect of different drugs on exercise-induced asthma. In preparation, cited from reference No 24.
27. Altounyan, R. E. C. (1967) Inhibition of experimental asthma by a new compound—disodium cromoglycate 'Intal'. *Acta Allergologica*, **22,** 487.
28. Pepys, J. and Hargreave, F. E. (1969) Disodium cromoglycate and induced asthma. *British Medical Journal*, **2,** 382.
29. Cox, J. S. G., Beach, J. E., Blair, A. M. J. N., Clarke, A. J., King, J., Lee, T. B., Loveday, D. E. E., Moss, G. F., Orr, T. S. C., Ritchie, Jean T., and Sheard, P. (1970) Disodium cromoglycate (INTAL). *Advances in Drug Research*, **5,** 115.
30. Brogden, R. N., Speight, T. M., and Avery, G. S., (1975) Sodium cromoglycate (cromolyn sodium): A review of its mode of action, pharmacology, therapeutic efficacy and use. *Drugs*, **7,** 164.
31. Brompton Hospital and Medical Research Council Collaborative Trial (1972) *British Medical Journal*, **4,** 383.

32. Walker, S. R., Evans, M. E., Richards, A. J., and Paterson, J. W. (1972) The fate of [^{14}C] disodium cromoglycate in man. *Journal of Pharmacy and Pharmacology*, **24**, 525.
33. Pepys, J. (1973) Disodium cromoglycate in clinical and experimental asthma. In *Asthma, Physiology, Immunopharmacology and Treatment*. (Ed. K. Frank Austen and Laurence M. Lichenstein). New York and London: Academic Press.
34. Silverman, M. and Andrea, T. (1972) The time-course of disodium cromoglycate in asthmatic children. *Archives of Diseases in Children* **47**, 419.
35. Silverman, M., König, P. and Godfrey, S. (1973) The use of serial exercise tests to assess the efficacy and duration of action of drugs in asthma. *Thorax*, **28**, 574.
36. Asano, T. and Asano, W. (1970) Results of long-term administration of Intal on infantile bronchial asthma (translation). *Japanese Journal of Paediatrics*, **23**, 105.
37. Bernstein, L., Siegal, S. C., Brandon, M. L., Brown, E. B., Evans, R. R., Feinberg, A. R., Friedlander, S., Krumhelz, R. A., Hadley, R. A., Handelman, N. I., Thurson, D., and Yamate, M. (1972) A controlled study of cromolyn sodium sponsored by the Drug Committee of the American Academy of Allergy. *Journal of Allergy and Clinical Immunology*, **50**, 235.
38. Collins-Williams, C., Chiu, A. W., Lamenza, C., Lewis-McKinley, C. A., Williams, H. and Levison, H. (1971) Treatment of bronchial asthma with disodium cromoglycate (Intal) in children. *Annals of Allergy*, **29**, 613.
39. Bedford, S. and Kuzemko, J. A., (1970) Treatment of asthmatic children for six months with disodium cromoglycate. *Clinical Paediatrics*, **9**, 719.
40. Dickson, W. (1970) A one year's trial of INTAL compound in 24 children with severe asthma. In *Disodium Cromoglycate in Allergic Airways Disease*, (Ed. Pepys & Frankland) London: Butterworths.
41. Hyde, J. S., Isenberg, P. D. and Floro, L. D. (1973) Short and long-term prophylaxis with cromolyn sodium in chronic asthma. *Chest*, **63**, 875.
42. Fox, Z. R., Brickman, H. F., Beaudy, P. H., Liddell, F. D. K., and Eisen, A. H. (1972) Response to disodium cromoglycate in children with chronic asthma. *Canadian Medical Association Journal*, **106**, 97.
43. Silverman, M., Connolly, N. M., Balfour-Lynn, L., and Godfrey, S. (1972) Long-term trial of disodium cromoglycate and isoprenaline in children with asthma. *British Medical Journal*, **3**, 378.
44. Jones, R. S. and Blackhall, M. I. (1970) Role of disodium cromoglycate in treatment of children's asthma. *Archives of Diseases in Childhood*, **45**, 49.
45. Chai, H., Molk, L., Falliers, C. J. and Miklich, D. (1971) Steroid sparing effects of disodium cromoglycate (DSC) in children with severe chronic asthma, In *Serafini New Concepts in Allergy and Clinical Immunology*, 385.
46. Engström, I. and Kraepelien, S. (1971) The coricosteroid sparing effect of disodium cromoglycate in children and adolescents with bronchial asthma. *Acta Allergologica*, **26**, 90.
47. Gelfand, M.L. (1951) Administration of cortisone by the aerosol method in the treatment of bronchial asthma, *New England Journal of Medicine*, **245**, 293.
48. Brockband, W. and Pengelly, C. D. R. (1958) Chronic asthma treated with powder inhalations of hydrocortisone and prednisolone. *Lancet*, **1**, 187.
49. Helm, W. H. and Heyworth, C. (1958) Inhalation of hydrocortisone acetate for bronchial asthma. *British Medical Journal*, **2**, 768.
50. Dennis, M. and Itkin, I. H. (1964) Effectiveness and complications of aerosol dexamethasone phosphate in severe asthma. *Journal of Allergy*, **35**, 70.
51. Novey, H. S. and Beall, G. (1965) Aerosolized steroids and induced Cushing's syndrome. *Archives of Internal Medicine*, **115**, 602.
52. McKenzie, A. W. and Stoughton, R. B. (1962) Method for comparing percutaneous absorption of steroids. *Archives of Dermatology*, **86**, 608.
53. Sparkes, C. G. (1974) Plasma cortisol levels in normal subjects after inhaled corticosteroids. *Postgraduate Medical Journal*, **50**, (Supplement 4), 9.
54. Friedman, Max, Frears, Janna and Crawley, Mary F. (1974) The effect of betamethasone valerate inhalation on the hypothalamic-pituitary-adrenal axis of normal

adults. *Postgraduate Medical Journal*, **50** (Supplement 4), 11.
55. Harris, D. M. (1975) The properties of beclomethasone dipropionate in men, *Postgraduate Medical Journal Supplement*, **51,** 20.
56. Dash, C. H. (1974) Some observations on the use of corticosteroid aerosols in asthma, *Postgraduate Medical Journal*, **50,** (Supplement 4), 25.
57. McAllen, M. K., Kochanowski, S. J. and Shaw, K. M. (1974) Steroid aerosols in asthma: An assessment of betamethasone valerate and a 12-month study of patients on maintenance treatment. *British Medical Journal*, **1,** 171.
58. Godfrey, S. (1974) Problems peculiar to the diagnosis and management of asthma in children. *The British Thoracic and Tuberculosis Association*, **4,** 1.
59. Dickson, W., Hall, C. E., Ellis, Mary and Horrocks, R. H. (1973) Beclomethasone dipropionate aerosol in childhood asthma. *Archives of Diseases in Childhood*, **48,** 671.
60. Godfrey, S. and König, P. (1974) Treatment of childhood asthma for 13 months and longer with beclomethasone dipropionate aerosol. *Archives of Diseases in Childhood*, **49,** 591.
61. Brown, H. M. and Storey, G. (1973) Beclomethasone dipropionate steroid aerosol in treatment of perennial allergic asthma in children. *British Medical Journal*, **3,** 161.
62. Brown, H. M. and Storey, G. (1975) Becotide in the treatment of allergic asthma. *Postgraduate Medical Journal Supplement*, **51,** 59.
63. Kuzemko, J. A. (1974) Growth velocity in children on oral corticosteroids and betamethasone valerate aerosol, *Postgraduate Medical Journal*, **50** (Supplement 4), 38.
64. Grant, I. W. B. (1975) Experience with beclomethasone dipropionate aerosol in treatment of chronic asthma. *Postgraduate Medical Journal Supplement*, **51,** 57.
65. Clark, T. J. H., Costello, J. F., and Souter C. A. (1975) The effects of beclomethasone dipropionate aerosol given in higher doses to patients with asthma. *Postgraduate Medical Journal Supplement*, **51,** 72.
66. Frears, J. F., Wilson, L. C. and Friedman, M. (1963) Betamethasone 17-valerate by aerosol in childhood asthma. *Archives of Diseases in Childhood*, **48,** 856.
67. Frears, J. F., Maizels, J. and Friedman, M. (1975) Unpublished data.
68. Taylor, B. and Norman, A. P. (1974) Betamethasone 17-valerate aerosol in children not on previous steroid therapy. *Postgraduate Medical Journal*, **40** (Supplement 4), 44.
69. Kuzemko, J. A., Bedford, S. Wilson, Lyn and Walker, S. R. (1974) A comparison of betamethasone valerate aerosol and sodium cromoglycate in children with reversible airways obstruction. *Postgraduate Medical Journal*, **50** (Supplement 4), 53.
70. Hiller, Elizabeth J. (1974) Sodium cromoglycate compared with betamethasone valerate in children. *Postgraduate Medical Journal*, **50** (Supplement 4), 58.
71. Friedman, Max and Frears, Janna. (1974) Hypothalamic-pituitary-adrenal function and growth in asthmatic children on long-term betamethasone valerate aerosol. *Postgraduate Medical Journal*, **50,** (Supplement 4), 33.
72. König, P., Jaffe, P. J. and Godfrey, S. (1974) The effect of corticosteroids on exercise-induced asthma. *Journal of Allergy and Clinical Immunology*, **54,** 14.
73. Heimlich, E. M., Strick, L. and Busser, R. J. (1966) An exercise response test in childhood asthma. *Journal of Allergy*, **37,** 103.
74. Hodgson, Shirley V., McPherson, Ann and Friedman, Max. (1974) The effect of betamethasone valerate aerosol on exercise-induced asthma in children. *Postgraduate Medical Journal*, **50** (Supplement 4), 69.
75. Poynter, D. and Spurling, N. W. and Ainge G. (1975) Toxicity trials with beclomethasone dipropionate in the dog with particular reference to the respiratory tract. *Postgraduate Medical Journal Supplement*, **51,** 27.
76. Thiringer, G., Eriksson, N., Malmberg, R., Svedmyr, N. and Zettergren, L. (1975) Bronchoscopic biopsies of bronchial mucosa before and after beclomethasone dipropionate therapy. *Postgraduate Medical Journal Supplement*, **51,** 30.
77. Andersson, E. and Smidt, C. M. (1974) An investigation of the bronchial mucous membrane after long term treatment with beclomethasone dipropionate (Becotide). *Acta Allergologica*, **29,** 354.
78. Milne, L. J. R. and Compton, G. K. (1974) Beclomethasone dipropionate and

oropharyngeal candidiasis. *British Medical Journal*, **3,** 797.
79. Friedman, Max (1975) Personal Communication.
80. Kuzemko, J. A. (1975) Personal Communication.
81. Campbell, I. A. (1975) Inhaled corticosteroids compared with oral prednisone in patients starting long term corticosteroid therapy for asthma. *Lancet*, **2,** 469.
82. Bainbridge, D., Hoare, M. V., McHardy, G. J. R. and Dash, C. H. (1975) A double-blind trial of salmefamol, a new bronchodilator. *Postgraduate Medical Journal*, **51,** 627.
83. Goldberg, R., Joffe, B. I., Bersohn, I., Van As, M., Krut, L., and Seftel, H. C. (1975) Metabolic responses to selective β-adrenergic stimulation in man. *Postgraduate Medical Journal*, **51,** 53.
84. Taylor, M. W., Gaddie, J., Murchison, L. E., and Palmer, K. N. V. (1976) Metabolic effects of oral salbutamol. *British Medical Journal*, **1,** 22.

Appendix

DRUGS OF VALUE IN ASTHMA

Group I Sympathomimetics

Drug	Presentation	Dose	Route of administration
Adrenaline	Solution, 1/1,000	0·1 to 0·5 ml	Subcutaneously
Ephedrine hydrate	Tablets, 15 mg	7·5 to 30 mg	Orally
Ethylnoradrenaline hydrochloride.	Solution, 1/500	up to 1·0 ml in 250 ml, diluent	Intravenously
Isoprenaline sulphate	Aerosol pressurised self-activated	0·08 mg/inhal.	Inhalation
Terbutaline sulphate	Tablets, 5mg	½ to 1	Orally
	Elixir, 0·3 mg/ml	5 to 15 ml t.d.s.	,,
	Aerosol, 0·2 mg/dose	1 puff, p.r.n.	Inhalation
	Solution, 0·5 mg/ml	0·25 ml (0·125 mg)	Subcutaneous
Orciprenaline sulphate	Tablets, 20 mg	½ to 1 tablet	Orally
	Syrup, 10 mg/5 ml	2·5 to 5 ml	Orally
	Solution, 0·5 mg/ml	½ to 1 ml	Subcutaneous
	Aerosol, 15 mg/ml, each dose 0·75 mg	1 puff	Inhalation
Salbutamol sulphate	Tablets, 2 and 4 mg	2 to 4 mg prn.	Orally
	Syrup, 2 mg/5 ml	2·5 to 10 ml p.r.n.	,,
	Respirator solution 1/200	0·25 to 2 ml	Nebuliser
	Aerosol, 0·1 mg/dose	1 to 2 puffs	Aerosol inhalation
Rimiterol	Aerosol only	1 to 2 puffs	Aerosol inhalation

Group II Xanthines

Drug	Presentation	Dose	Route of administration
Theophylline	Elixir, 80 mg/15 ml.	0·5 ml/kg weight t.d.s.	Orally
Aminophylline (Theophylline-ethylenediamine)	Suppositories, 50 and 100 mg	50 to 100 mg	Rectally
,,	Solution,	15 mg/kg weight per 24 hours. 4 mg/kg weight as maximum single dose	Intravenously
Choline theophyllinate	Tablets, 100 mg	1 t.d.s. in older children	Orally
	Syrup, 50 mg/5 ml	2.5 to 5 ml t.d.s.	Orally

Group III Antihistamines

Drug	Presentation	Dose	Route of administration
Tripolidine hydrochloride	Tablets, 2·5 mg	½ to 1, t.d.s.	Orally
	Elixir, 1 mg/5 ml	2·5 to 10 ml	„
Diphenhydramine hydrochloride	Elixir, 12·5 mg/5 ml	2 to 5 ml	„
Chlorpheniramine maleate	Syrup, 2 mg/5 ml	1 to 5 ml	„
Meclozine hydrochloride	Elixir, 12·5 mg/5 ml	2·5 to 5 ml b.d.	„
	(Also useful in motion sickness)		
Mepyramine maleate	Elixir, 25 mg/5 ml	12·5 to 50 mg	„
Promethazine hydrochloride	Tablets, 10 mg	1 twice daily	„
	Elixir, 5 mg/5 ml	2·5 to 10 ml b.d.	„
	Injection, 25 mg/ml		Subcutaneously
Clemastine	Tablets, 1 mg	½ to 1; 1 or 2 per day	Orally
	Paed. Liq. 0·25 mg per 5 ml	2·5 to 10 ml	„
Trimepramine tartrate	Tablets, 10 mg	½ tablet, max.	„
	Syrup, 7·5 mg/5 ml	2·5 to 7·5 ml	„
(Care should be exercised, as some children become unrousable, even up to 36 hours).			

Group IV Antibiotics

Drug	Presentation	Dose	Route of administration
Penicillin, G and Benzyl	Powder for soln.	¼ to 2 million units	Intramuscularly or intravenously
Penicillin V	Tablets, 125 and 250 mg	1 to 2, 2–4 times a day	Orally
	Suspension, 125 mg per 5 ml	5 to 10 ml	„
	Capsules, as tablets		
Ampicillin	Capsules, 250 mg	1 capsule 4/day	„
	Injections, 100, 250, 500 mg	100/250 mg	Intramuscularly, or intravenously
	Paed. Tablets, 125 mg	1–2 4/day	Orally
	Syrup, 125 mg/5 ml	2·5 to 10 ml	„
	„ Forte, 250 mg/5 ml	„	„
Amoxacillin	As for Ampicillin		
Cloxacillin	As for Ampicillin Potent against staphylococci		
Flucloxacillin	„		

Group IV Antibiotics—*contd.*

Drug	Presentation	Dose	Route of administration
Erythromycin stearate	As for Ampicillin. Of use especially in penicillin-sensitive patients. Spectrum as Benzyl Penicillin.		
Trimethoprim-sulphamethoxazole	Tablets. Dose ½ to 1 tablet b.d. Orally Paed. Suspension 2·5 to 10 ml b.d. Orally Available in a wide range of preparations, singly and in various combinations.		
tetracyclines	Can be of value in the older child. Must not be given to young children owing to the risk of staining the teeth.		

Group V Sodium cromoglycate

Drug	Presentation	Dose	Route of administration
Intal	Capsules, 20 mg yellow and white	1 to 6/day.	Inhalation by Spinhaler
Rynacrom	Capsules, 10 mg (pink)	4 to 12/day.	Nasal insufflator

Group VI Oral corticosteroids.

Drug	Presentation	Dose	Route of administration
Prednisolone or Prednisone	Tablets, 1 and 5 mg	As indicated in text.	Orally
	(Solution for injection)	50 to 200 mg	Intravenously

There are many other corticosteroids, including—
hydrocortisone (not used orally), dexamethasone, betamethasone, etc.
They are used, not only orally, but also as topical applications, either singly or combined with an antibiotic.

Group VII Corticotrophins

Drug	Presentation	Dose	Route of administration
ACTH,	Gel for injection, 25 or 40 i.u./ml	10 to 40 units as indicated	deep intra-muscularly.
Synacthen (Tetracosactrin)	Vials, 5 ml 0·2 mg/ml	0·125–0·25 mg	intramuscular
Synacthen depot	0·5 mg/1 ml.	,,	,,

Group VIII Aerosol Steroids

Drug	Presentation	Dose	Route administration
Becotide—beclomethasone diproprionate	Pressurised aerosol. 200 doses, of 50 μg/dose	2 puffs 2 to 4/day	Inhalation
Bextasol betamethasone-17-valerate	Pressurised aerosol. 200 doses, of 100 μg/dose	"	"

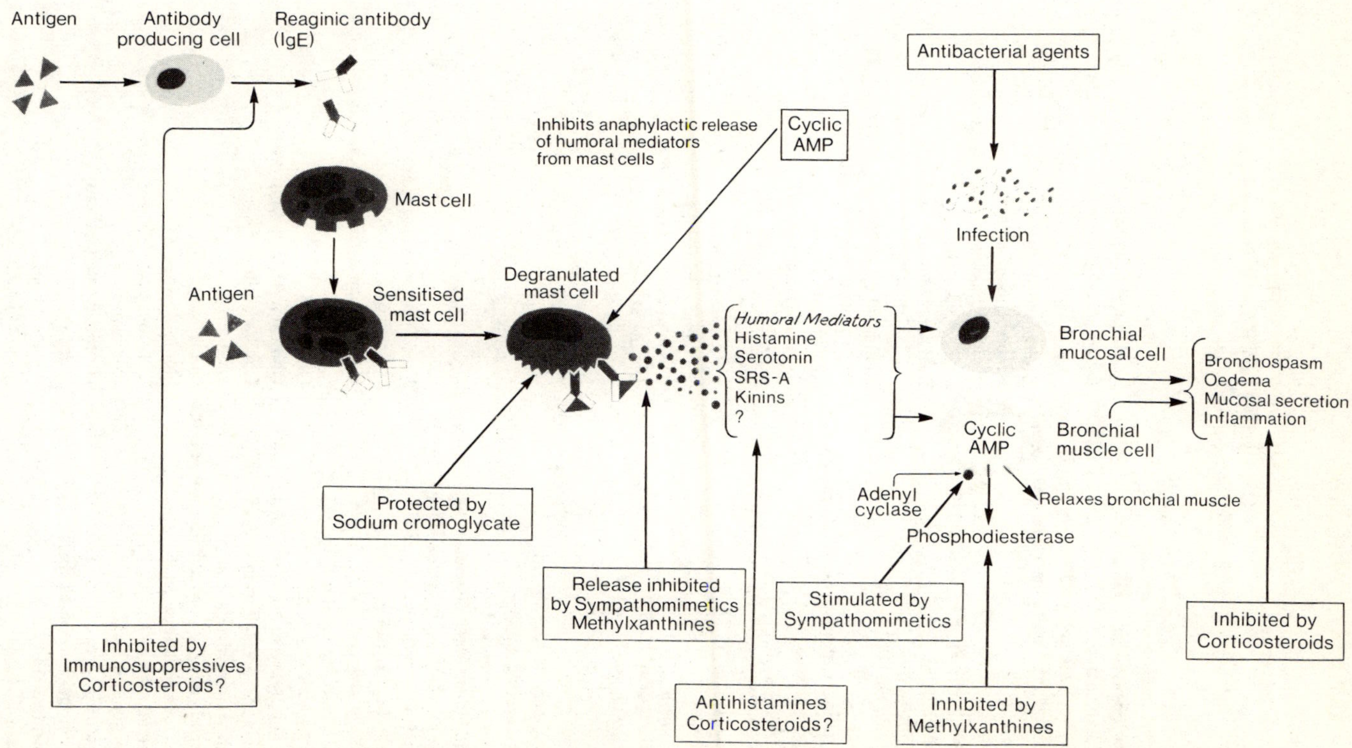

Schematic representation of pharmacological mechanisms in asthma showing site and mode of action of antiasthmatic drugs (simplified)

Index